# Contents

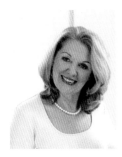

The first thing you must do before you start on this or any diet, is to check the state of your health with your doctor. You will certainly lose weight on this diet, and you'll probably find other good things (such as a drop in blood pressure, or better heart health) have happened to your body, so your doctor will be able to note these changes when you check in again after completing the diet.
Read through the next few pages carefully, so you can prepare to embark on this diet. Work out a moderate exercise program to suit yourself and your diet partner; don't push yourself too hard, let your body adjust gently to the diet. Walking briskly for 30 minutes every day will certainly help you in every way.
These recipes are easy, filling, practical, inexpensive, tasty and quick. Most of the meals take less than 30 minutes to prepare, and all the ingredients can be found in any supermarket. Weigh yourself once a week – you'll be amazed at the results and how good you feel. We think this wonder diet ticks all the boxes for our modern lifestyle.

*Pamela Clark*

Food Director

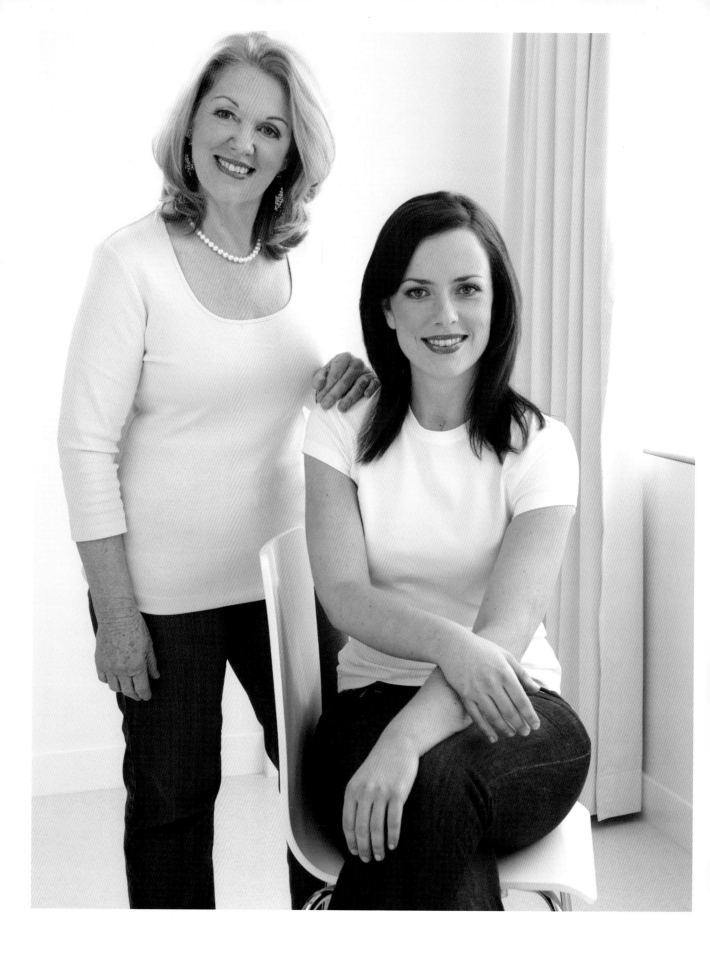

# The dieters

**INTRODUCING PAMELA CLARK AND SARAH SCHWIKKARD,** the Test Kitchen guinea pigs. Pamela, Test Kitchen Director, and Sarah, Test Kitchen Food Editor, embarked on a mission to try out the 21-day diet in order to get their bodies ship-shape in time for another hot Sydney summer.

Working weeks jam-packed with functions, meetings and taste-testing rules Pamela's food routine. Like most Baby Boomers out there, her weekends revolve around tending to grandparent duties, socialising with family and friends, gardening, and the never-ending list of things to do around the house; this hectic schedule means that there is little time left to fuss over healthy eating. Pamela felt that it was time to get some balance back in her life, and what better opportunity to do it than when a diet cookbook is being developed at work.

Representing Generation Y, Sarah decided that it was time to lose the lumps and bumps she'd acquired from tasting food non-stop in the Test Kitchen. Partial to sugary foods, champagne and "grazing", Sarah's eating habits were in need of a serious shake-up. For this serial dieter, the thought of eating three healthy meals each day was rather confronting; she had to accept that weekends filled with indulgent dinners and drinks were about to become a thing of the past. Sarah admitted that part of her problem was her inability to be disciplined with routine; it was time for her to learn to restrain, and retrain, her body in order to kill the sugar cravings – once and for all.

Pamela lost 5.5kg in the 21 days and Sarah was not far behind with 5kg off her frame. They both found the diet so easy to stick to that they repeated it – again with fabulous results. The (former) guinea pigs are now ready to face summer feeling revitalised, fresh and fantastic.

**BODY MASS INDEX** (BMI), is a creation of the World Health Organisation, and is used by medical professionals worldwide to determine weight classifications. It is calculated by dividing a person's weight in kilograms by their height in metres squared. For example, a person who is 1.7m tall and weighs 70kg would have a BMI of 24; this is considered a healthy BMI. A BMI of 25-29 is classified as overweight; a BMI of more than 30 is classified as obese.

A healthy-eating plan that is balanced, low-in-fat but high-in-taste: sound impossible? Well, it's not. We've developed a diet that doesn't mirror any of the "fad" diets on the market today; our key to success is a menu plan with less than 20g fat per day. Average Australians consume between 50g to 60g fat per day; by reducing this intake by more than half, it is obvious why our diet is foolproof. Whether you want to lose weight for medical reasons, for a special upcoming event or just for your own wellbeing, this diet is for you.

## ATTACK THE FAT

Fat is not our enemy. However, with obesity rates in Australia at an all-time high, it is important that we educate ourselves about fat, and recognise the difference between "good" and "bad" fats. You may have heard of saturated fats and trans fats: these are "bad" fats. Found in fatty meats, commercial cakes and deep-fried takeaway food, "bad" fats increase the risk of heart disease and contribute to high blood cholesterol. "Good" fats, like polyunsaturated fats and monounsaturated fats, are abundant in oils such as sunflower and olive, as well as salmon, tuna, nuts, lean meats and seeds; these fats can help lower blood cholesterol and reduce the risk of heart disease.

## 21 DAYS OF DISCIPLINE

If Pamela and Sarah can do this diet, anyone can. True to Women's Weekly style, the recipes we've developed (and tested to perfection) are easy-to-follow, there are no hard-to-find ingredients and, best of all, the diet is incredibly inexpensive; losing weight doesn't have to make your pockets lighter, just your body! We believe that it's imperative to eat in order to trim down; by eating three meals and two snacks per day, for 21 days, you'll find that you lose weight in a fashion that is good for your body – and the weight will stay off.

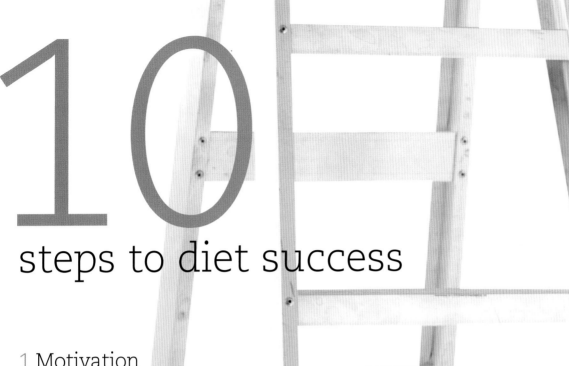

# 10
## steps to diet success

1 Motivation
2 Planning
3 Exercise
4 Water
5 Scales
6 Sleep
7 Special occasions
8 Support
9 Shopping
10 Maintenance

**FACTS ABOUT THE
WONDER DIET**
This diet is based on the
Healthy Eating Pyramid
and follows the Australian
Dietary Guidelines.
**This is a serious weight-loss
diet that will supply your
body with around 4000kJ
(1000 cal) per day.**
The diet is for two people,
based on three meals to be
shared and two snacks per
person, per day.

# Motivation

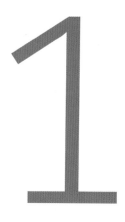

### ARE YOU READY TO LOSE WEIGHT?

There's no point embarking on a lifestyle change unless you're mentally
prepared. It's vital that you've thought carefully about why you want to
lose weight and, most importantly, who you're losing weight for (the
answer should be you). Without the commitment, the drive and the
passion to achieve results for yourself with this diet, it will be a challenge
to be successful.

### WRITE A LIST

If you've recognised that you need a change, whether it's because your
jeans don't zip up anymore, you're short of breath when you chase the
kids around the park, or the photos from last Christmas make you cringe,
then it's time to be pro-active and make a change. A good way to start is to
write a list of things you like about yourself, and a list of things you're not
too happy with; this will help clear your mind, and give you focus to start
the diet.

### SET A GOAL FOR YOURSELF

Perhaps it's a dress that you haven't been able to zip up for years, or you
want to tone up your legs for some new summer shorts, by setting a goal,
it gives you something to work towards; write it down on a piece of paper
and stick it somewhere visible – like on your computer at work or on your
mirror in the bathroom. Every time you look at it, it'll give you motivation,
and remind you why you're doing the diet – for yourself.

## FACTS ABOUT THE WONDER DIET

The diet is low in fat, it is below 20g fat per day; the average Australian eats 60g fat per day.
The diet is low in sugar, except for the natural sugars found in fruit.
The diet is moderate in iron; citrus juice (vitamin C) is used in the recipes for flavour and to help iron absorption.
This is a low-sodium (salt) diet so we've used fresh herbs for flavouring. Herbs also contain vitamins, minerals and anti-oxidants.

### STOCKING UP

Out of sight, out of mind: this saying goes hand-in-hand with diet mentality. If you don't have any junk food in your cupboard, you won't be tempted to eat it. Fill your fridge, freezer and pantry with healthy foods, so even if you feel like a midnight snack, you'll be munching on a carrot stick, rather than a bag of chips.

### ORGANISING YOUR LIFE

Not only do you need to be motivated and committed, it's paramount that you're organised and prepared for this diet. By being 100% prepared, it means that you don't give yourself a chance to slip back into bad habits. For example, if you know that Mondays are notoriously busy for you, then make dinner for Monday on Sunday night and pop it in the fridge or freezer. This means that you avoid coming home from work on Monday, tired and hungry, and reaching for the phone to order a pizza. You can always get your family involved, too; the recipes in this diet are all kid-friendly – if you're having a tuna salad for lunch, then so can they. Make a double quantity of the recipe and you'll find that you halve the time you spend in the kitchen.

### SWAPPING DAYS

Feel free to swap days around on the diet to suit your lifestyle. For example, if you look at the menu for Day 6 and think that you would rather have the food from Day 11 instead, then just swap them around. Same goes for the snacks – feel free to chop and change. By making changes like this, you're making life easier for yourself, and you'll find it easier to stick to the diet.

# Planning

# Exercise

3

## SWEAT IT OUT

Whether you like it or not, exercise is integral to weight loss. We're not talking about running marathons here, just regular, moderate exercise. Not only will exercising help you lose weight and tone your body, but it makes you feel good, too. Why? Well, when you exercise, your brain releases endorphins – nature's "happy pill". It's certainly a cheap and easy way to get a smile on your dial. So, if you're feeling a bit flat or you've had a bad day, the best thing you can do is go and do some exercise – it'll make you feel better in no time.

## MAKE TIME FOR EXERCISE

Morning, noon or night, any time is a good time for fitness. If you're not a morning person, then how about taking the dog for a walk at sunset. Or, if you always work late at night, then get up half an hour earlier and put your exercise gear on. Lunchtime exercise is also a great way to fit it into your day; rather than eating lunch at your desk, walk down to a park bench and eat it there. Not only do you get a bit of exercise before you eat, but you also get a good dose of fresh air before you return to the office. Weekends are always a good time to get fit; instead of going out for coffee and cake, get a group of friends together and go for a long walk.

## INCIDENTAL EXERCISE

There are lots of ways to fit "incidental exercise" into your day – this is exercise that isn't formal exercise, but it's all these extra bits of activity that you do that can make a difference. For example, take the stairs instead of the lift, park your car far away from the supermarket, or even better, leave your car at home and walk to the shops instead.

DID YOU KNOW that if you eat a 50g piece of milk chocolate, you need to walk briskly for over 60 minutes to burn off the kilojoules?

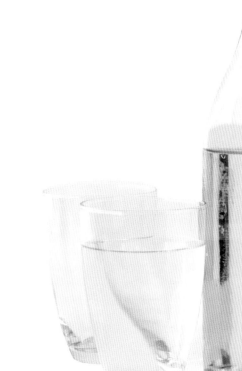

**FACTS ABOUT THE
WONDER DIET**
Drink at least 2 litres
of water every day;
include tea, coffee
etc., in this count.
We suggest you avoid
alcohol-based drinks
while you're on this diet.

# Water

4

## HYDRATION

It is paramount that you keep your body hydrated when you do the diet.
Not enough water can do a number of things to you – apart from the
obvious, and most severe, dehydration, a lack of water can make you
tired and also give you headaches. By drinking at least 2 litres of water
a day, you'll be keeping your body and mind in line. Water also aids with
satiety (feeling full), and a glass of water is certainly better for you than
a chocolate biscuit.

## A SPARKLE IN YOUR EYES

It may sound too good to be true, but by drinking lots of water, you're
helping your skin, hair and eyes to look great. People who drink a lot
of water generally have a clear complexion, shiny hair and a sparkle
in their eyes.

# Scales

**5**

**WEIGHTS AND MEASURES**

The recipes in this diet have been carefully measured and triple-tested, so it is important to use the weights that we've given in the recipes, to ensure that you are getting the nutrition we intended. Take the guesswork out and invest in kitchen scales if you don't own them already; scales come in handy for weighing meat, poultry and seafood.

Flavour-enhancers like chilli, mustard, herbs and spices can be used with abandon as they contain a negligible amount of fat and kilojoules. Take care when using cooking-oil spray; a 1-second spray of oil is measured as 1g of fat, so apply sparingly.

**WEIGH-IN**

Weighing yourself every day will not give you a true reflection of your weight-loss; weight can fluctuate from day-to-day. It helps to be consistent with what you wear when you weigh-in, too – preferably weigh yourself naked to give a true indication of what you weigh, otherwise wear something lightweight. It's also good to weigh yourself at the same time, for example, 7am every Monday morning; and make sure you use the same set of scales every time.

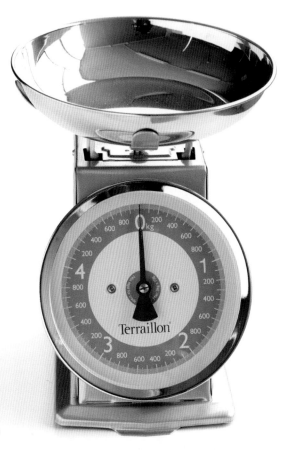

### SLEEP WELL, LOOK SWELL

It's important that you look after your body when you are on a diet. By depriving yourself of sleep, your energy stores become depleted and staying awake during the day becomes a real struggle. Keep your energy levels high and mood positive by getting at least eight hours sleep a night. You'll look better for it, too, with no tell-tale signs of tiredness, like dark circles under your eyes. A good night's sleep is also necessary to give your body time to repair; the human body is constantly working, using the nutrients it collects from your food to strengthen and recharge your muscles.

### NIGHT-TIME WEIGHT-LOSS

Not only does a good rest give you energy, but it also helps you lose weight. While you sleep, your body burns calories (yes, it's true!); on average, you burn about 3.8kJ/0.9 calories per minute of sleep – there's no better excuse to get some shut-eye.

### STOP SNORING

A very common problem among men and women alike, snoring, and sleep apnoea, is prevalent predominantly in overweight middle-aged males. Alcohol, caffeine, sleep deprivation and late-night eating are top things to avoid if you'd like a night without the disruption caused by snoring.

### RELAX AND UNWIND

For many of us, falling asleep after a stressful, busy day is often with great effort; however, if you go to bed relaxed, chances are that you will sleep well. Drinking non-caffeinated herbal teas before you sleep, and burning aromatherapy oils in your bedroom, both assist in helping you relax before you go to bed. By creating a warm, soothing environment where you sleep, you will wake up feeling refreshed and ready for another day.

# Sleep

## STRATEGIC EATING

Holidays, birthday parties, work functions, dinner parties ... the list can go on and on – these are all events where over-eating is notorious. Being on a diet doesn't mean that you have to avoid attending special occasions, you simply need to make smart eating choices, ensuring that you don't become the pig of the party. If you're dining out, don't be shy to ask the waiter if you can alter the meal slightly to suit your dietary needs; for example, ask for sauces and dressings to be served on the side, grill fish instead of frying – it's all about strategic eating.

## RESIST AND WIN

Nibbles and treats need to be resisted in order to achieve diet success; things like garlic bread at restaurants, chips and dips at parties and ice-cream at the movies are all laden with fat and sugar, and only provide temporary satisfaction. You're far better off to ignore these foods and enjoy your main meal, rather than filling up on the unnecessary side-dishes.

## SLOWLY DOES IT

If you choose to have a glass of wine at a function, drink it slowly, rather than guzzling glass after glass. Alcohol, in particular beer, contains a lot of kilojoules so opt for a dry white wine or champagne, if you can. The best option however, is to drink water; sparkling mineral water is surprisingly rewarding, not to mention a far cheaper option than alcohol.

## CUT THE CAKE

This diet isn't based on torture and guilt; there may be times when you are dying for a taste of chocolate or something a little naughty, so, if the birthday cake looks too good to resist, go mad, have a tiny piece. Just bear in mind, that for any extra kilojoules you consume, you need to do extra exercise to compensate.

7

**FACTS ABOUT THE WONDER DIET**
You can eat the bran and cranberry muesli (p32) every day of this diet instead of following our breakfast suggestions. Swap whole days around to suit your tastes in food, but don't mix and match lunches and dinners. Swap lunches for dinners (on the same day) if it suits your lifestyle better.

# Special occasions

# Support

### STRESS RELIEVERS

It makes a great deal of difference if you have a "support team" by your side during the diet. Whether it's your partner, your next-door neighbour or a group of girls from work, a little bit of support goes a long way. There will be easy days, as well as hard days on the journey; sharing your thoughts, problems and excitement with the "team" will help decrease any stress or doubt you may be feeling. If you know you have a problem with discipline, having a group of people you feel you can turn to can be a fantastic way to ensure you don't slip back into old eating habits.

### POSITIVE ATTITUDE

The art of positive thinking plays a big role in reaching goals in life, and achieving success in the diet is no exception. You need to retain a positive frame of mind throughout the diet; doing the diet should be a positive experience, and you should feel proud of yourself for committing to it. Be confident about your decision to change your lifestyle, and you will find that others will share in your confidence, too. Ignore any negativity that is directed at you in relation to your weight-loss.

### DEAR DIARY

Another easy way to keep yourself on track is to write a journal – doing so helps you remain accountable for your actions; like they say, if you cheat, you're only cheating yourself. Every day, jot down how you felt about the meals you ate, the exercise you did, record your weight loss and any thoughts you want to share with yourself. As the days go by, you can flick back and reflect on the progress you have made.

**FACT ABOUT THE WONDER DIET**
If your diet partner is not on this diet to lose weight, they can add more protein and carbs.

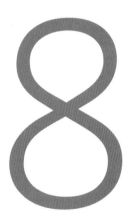

# Shopping

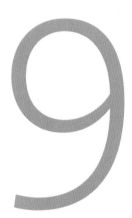

**FACTS ABOUT THE WONDER DIET**
This is a high-fibre diet; it's rich in vegetables and fruit. There are 5 servings of vegetables and 2 of fruit per day. The diet is high in calcium, achieved by including low-fat dairy products every day. There are three servings of seafood (fresh and canned) per week.

**SOUND STRUCTURE**
The best way to tackle the supermarket is to write a shopping list – and stick to it. We've made shopping even easier for you, by ensuring that there are no ingredients used in the 21-day diet plan that can't be found in a regular supermarket. By going to the shops with a structured list, you have no need to venture down the junk-food aisle. Shopping with a list in hand is efficient, and most likely to be cost-effective, too.

**SHOP FULL**
Avoid shopping on an empty stomach; if you're hungry, you're more likely to be tempted to buy the foods that you shouldn't eat.

**NUTRITION KNOW-HOW**
Checking the nutrition information panel on food labels is a good way to educate yourself about what you're eating. It's an interesting way to learn about the composition of different foods; information about energy (kilojoules), protein, total fat, saturated fat, carbohydrate, sugar and sodium are displayed on this panel. Be wary of food labelled with claims of being "low-fat", "low-joule" or "low-salt" – this is sometimes just a marketing strategy employed to catch out ignorant consumers.

**IT PAYS TO HAVE TIME**
Although not always possible to achieve, it's beneficial to go grocery shopping when it's not too busy, i.e., avoid Saturday mornings and late-night trading if you can. You want to be calm and relaxed when shopping to avoid having to make hasty decisions about what you put in your trolley.

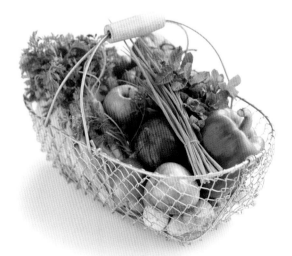

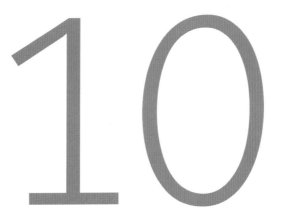

**A+ FOR EFFORT**

If you want to sustain your weight loss, you need to put in effort. After being disciplined for 21 days and achieving fantastic results, you don't want to un-do all the hard work you've done; identify your vices, whether it's pizzas, chocolate bars or thick shakes, and steer clear.

**INCREASE YOUR INTAKE**

Once you've finished the diet, if you'd like to maintain the weight you are at, you can increase your kilojoule intake, as long as you continue to exercise. There is however, no reason why you can't repeat the diet, like Pamela and Sarah successfully did.

**EMOTIONAL EATING**

Be happy to eat, don't eat to be happy – it is crucial that you don't binge-eat or make poor food choices to compensate for any emotional imbalance, otherwise you will find it difficult to maintain your ideal weight. The best thing you can do for yourself if you're feeling down is to put on your exercise gear, and get some fresh air.

**BREAKFAST FUEL**

Eating breakfast doesn't stop after the 21-day diet; maintaining your weight will be a lot easier if you continue to eat three full meals per day. If you don't have time to cook or bake your breakfast every morning, you can always make a large batch of our bran and cranberry muesli (see recipe, p32), as a stand-by breakfast saviour.

**SMILE**

Remember who you're doing this for: you. Be positive, be proud and be happy that you're pro-active and making a better life for yourself.

# Maintenance

# Day 1 Menu

melon trio with fresh lime and yogurt | dijon chicken and salad wrap | spiced lamb cutlets with coriander pumpkin

# melon trio with fresh lime and yogurt

**preparation time** 10 minutes **serves** 2
**nutritional count per serving** 0.8g total fat
(0.1g saturated fat); 573kJ (137 cal);
25.4g carbohydrate; 5.3g protein; 2.6g fibre

200g rockmelon, halved lengthways
200g honeydew melon, halved lengthways
200g watermelon, quartered crossways
2 tablespoons lime juice
½ cup (140g) skim-milk fruit-flavoured yogurt

1 Serve melons drizzled with juice, then dolloped with yogurt.

**Sarah's diary**
*I woke up this morning quite excited about starting the diet. Wasn't disappointed at all with breakfast – it was yum. I was flat-out all morning so lunch was a welcome reprieve...it took me back to school days with the simple chicken and salad combo. Managed to get through the day without dipping my hand into the cookie jar (a first). I hope this motivation and discipline continues.*

**Pamela's diary**
*The first day of any diet can be a bit tricky for me; it always takes me three days to get into a routine. On the first day, I go through various stages, first feeling enthusiastic, then second, thinking, maybe I should start the following day, or even the following week. Procrastination should be my middle name. Anyway, here we go.*

Choose whatever yogurt flavour you like; passionfruit flavour goes well with these fruits. Did you know melons are one of the best of all fruits. They're gentle on your digestive system and full of hydrating water and minerals.

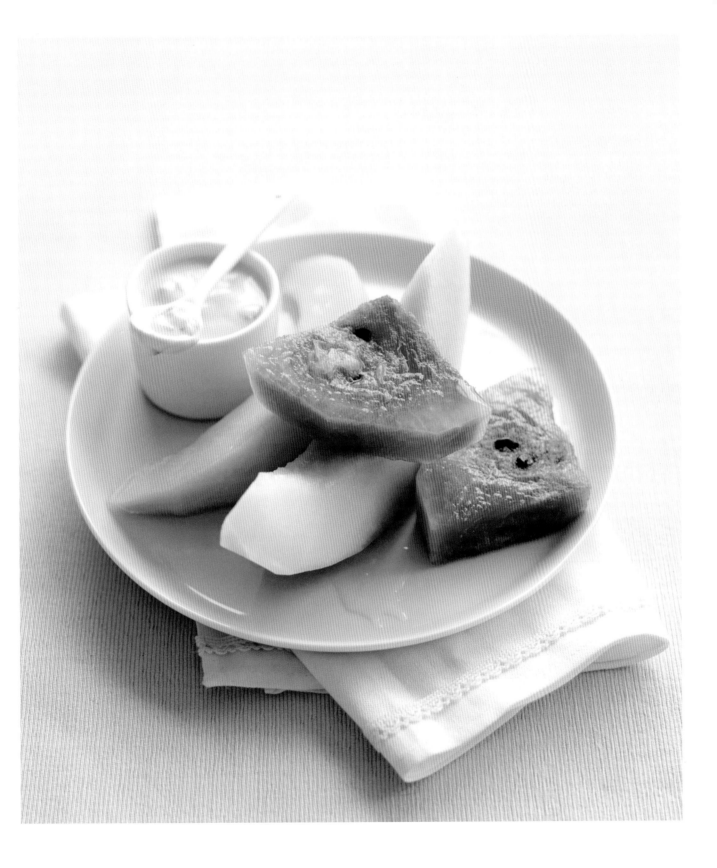

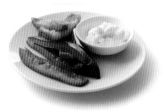

snack 1 small
red capsicum with
1 tablespoon low-fat
cottage cheese

If you're one of those people
who can't eat raw capsicum,
then swap this snack for
another in this book.
The wraps can be made in the
morning to take to work; you
can use any leafy greens you
like in place of the spinach.

# dijon chicken and salad wrap

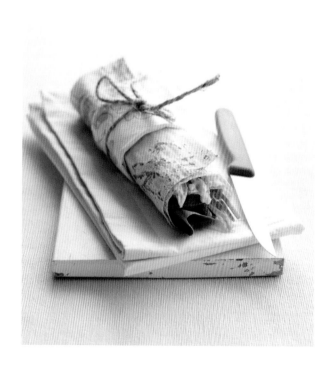

200g chicken breast fillet
cooking-oil spray
1 tablespoon skim-milk natural yogurt
1 teaspoon dijon mustard
2 rye mountain bread wraps (60g)
20g baby spinach
1 small tomato (90g), sliced thinly
1 small carrot (70g), grated coarsely

1  Spray chicken with cooking oil; cook chicken in
heated small frying pan. Cool; shred coarsely.
2  Combine chicken in medium bowl with yogurt
and mustard.
3  Divide chicken mixture between wraps; top with
remaining ingredients. Roll to enclose filling.

preparation time 10 minutes
cooking time 15 minutes  serves 2
nutritional count per serving  3.8g total fat
(0.7g saturated fat); 932kJ (223 cal);
17.9g carbohydrate; 27.4g protein; 3.2g fibre

# spiced lamb cutlets with coriander pumpkin

200g butternut pumpkin, peeled, cut into 1cm pieces
125g can chickpeas, rinsed, drained
½ cup (60g) frozen baby peas
2 tablespoons fresh coriander leaves
4 french-trimmed lamb cutlets (200g)
2 teaspoons curry powder
cooking-oil spray
⅓ cup (80ml) light coconut milk
2 tablespoons chicken stock
1 clove garlic, crushed

1  Preheat oven to 200°C/180°C fan-forced.
2  Roast pumpkin in small, shallow baking dish, uncovered, 10 minutes. Add chickpeas and peas; cook, uncovered, about 5 minutes or until pumpkin is tender. Remove from oven; sprinkle with coriander.
3  Meanwhile, sprinkle lamb with curry powder. Spray lamb with cooking oil. Cook lamb in heated medium frying pan; remove from pan.
4  Add coconut milk, stock and garlic to same pan, bring to the boil, stirring; remove from heat.
5  Serve pumpkin mixture and lamb drizzled with coconut sauce.

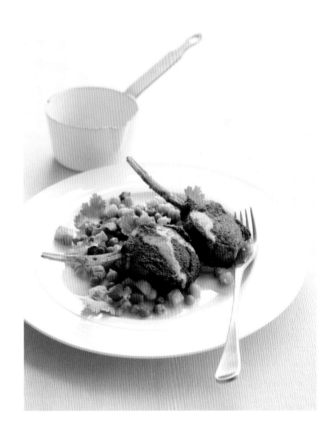

We used a mild curry powder for flavour but use what you like. Freeze any leftover coconut milk and store it in user-friendly portions for future meals.

**preparation time** 15 minutes
**cooking time** 15 minutes  **serves** 2
**nutritional count per serving**  9.3g total fat
(5.7g saturated fat); 978kJ (234 cal);
16.6g carbohydrate; 18.2g protein; 5.4g fibre

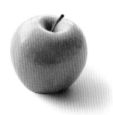

snack 1 small apple

# Day 2 Menu

cheesy corn on rye | potato, tuna and egg salad | chilli con carne

## cheesy corn on rye

preparation time 5 minutes
cooking time 30 seconds serves 2
nutritional count per serving 4.4g total fat
(1.7g saturated fat); 1120kJ (268 cal);
42.2g carbohydrate; 10.6g protein; 7.2g fibre

310g can corn kernels, rinsed, drained
2 tablespoons low-fat ricotta cheese
40g baby spinach leaves
2 slices rye bread (90g), toasted

1  Heat corn in medium bowl in microwave oven on HIGH
(100%) for about 30 seconds; stir in cheese and spinach.
2  Serve toast topped with corn mixture.

### Sarah's diary

*Got up at the crack of dawn
to go for a walk – I couldn't
believe the number of people
and dogs out and about at
that time. Absolutely loved
breakfast, was quick to
prepare and corn is one of
my faves. The exercise
must've got my metabolism
moving because I devoured
lunch in a flash. Dinner
consumed while watching
the news – trying to eat a
bit earlier than usual. My
housemates were most
impressed (and perhaps
shocked) that I didn't take
them up on their offer of
chocolate cake for dessert.*

### Pamela's diary

*I woke up hungry this
morning, and not feeling
energetic enough to go for
a walk. I must 'fess up to
having a small glass of
white wine with the family
last night, just to be
sociable. All three meals
today were filling and tasty,
but we also had a lot of food
to be tasted in the Test
Kitchen – it's not easy being
on a diet around here.*

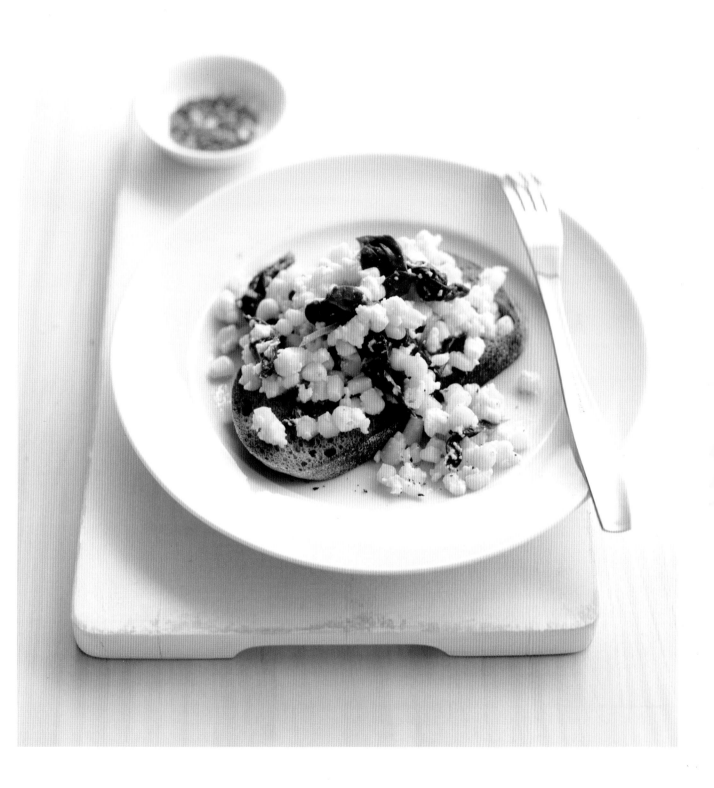

Toast is best "done" on one side only for this kind of topping.

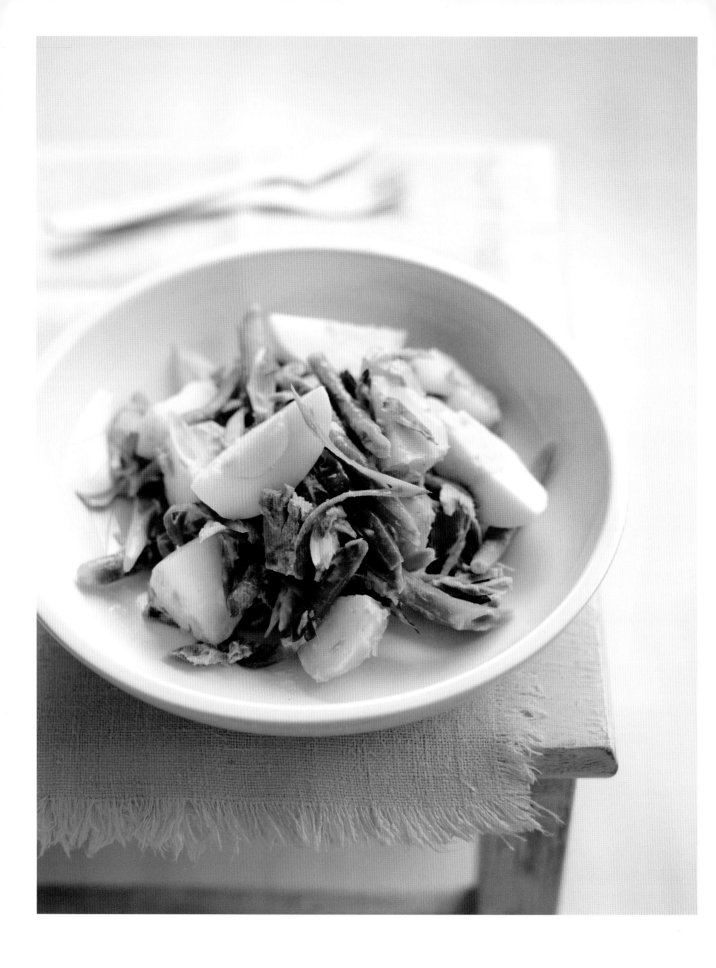

Make sure you prick the potatoes all over with a fork if you're cooking them in the microwave oven.
Salad can be made the night before – keep it in the fridge.

# potato, tuna and egg salad

**preparation time** 5 minutes
**cooking time** 10 minutes  **serves** 2
**nutritional count per serving**  2.5g total fat
(2.4g saturated fat); 1150kJ (275 cal);
18.9g carbohydrate; 30.7g protein; 3.9g fibre

6 baby new potatoes (240g)
100g green beans, trimmed, halved crossways
2 tablespoons skim-milk natural yogurt
1 teaspoon finely grated lemon rind
2 teaspoons lemon juice
185g can tuna in springwater, drained, flaked
3 green onions, sliced finely
1 tablespoon coarsely chopped fresh flat-leaf parsley
2 hard-boiled eggs, halved

1  Boil, steam or microwave potatoes and beans, separately, until tender; drain, cool.
2  Meanwhile, make dressing by combining yogurt, rind and juice in medium bowl.
3  Quarter potatoes; add to dressing with tuna, onion and parsley, stir to combine. Serve salad topped with egg.

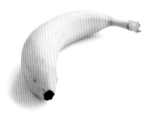

snack 1 small banana

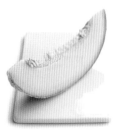

snack 200g rockmelon

# chilli con carne

**preparation time** 10 minutes
**cooking time** 30 minutes  **serves** 2
**nutritional count per serving**  7.9g total fat
(2.9g saturated fat); 1586kJ (378 cal);
43.5g carbohydrate; 28.6g protein; 8.3g fibre

⅓ cup (65g) brown rice
cooking-oil spray
1 small brown onion (80g), chopped finely
1 clove garlic, crushed
180g lean beef mince
1 teaspoon ground cumin
1 teaspoon dried chilli flakes
400g can diced tomatoes
2 tablespoons tomato paste
½ cup (125ml) beef stock
125g can four bean mix, rinsed, drained
2 tablespoons skim-milk natural yogurt
¼ cup coarsely chopped fresh flat-leaf parsley

1  Cook rice in medium saucepan of boiling water until
tender; drain.
2  Meanwhile, spray medium frying pan with cooking oil;
cook onion and garlic over heat, stirring, until onion softens.
Add beef and spices; cook, stirring, until beef is browned.
3  Add undrained tomatoes, paste and stock; bring to a
boil. Reduce heat; simmer, covered, 10 minutes. Uncover;
simmer about 10 minutes or until mixture thickens
slightly. Stir in beans.
4  Serve rice and chilli con carne topped with yogurt.
Sprinkle with parsley.

This is a great recipe (both
the rice and the mince
mixture) to cook in large
batches, ready to freeze
in user-friendly portions.
Freeze any leftover
tomato paste or stock.

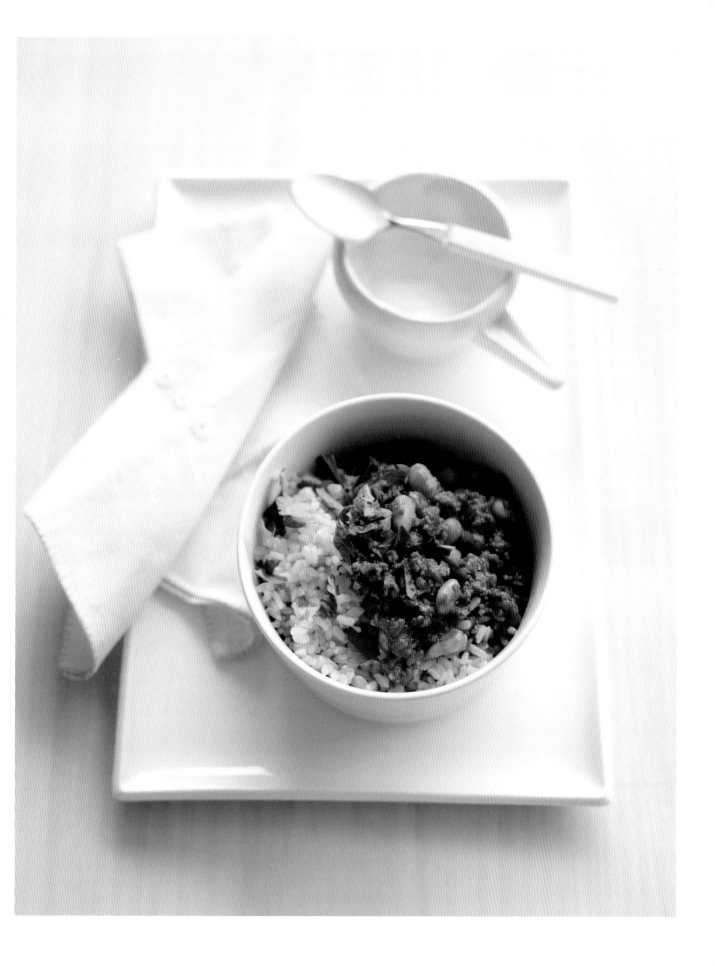

# Day 3 Menu

mango lassi | roast beef and coleslaw on rye | sumac fish with couscous salad

# mango lassi

**preparation time** 10 minutes  **serves** 2
**nutritional count per serving**  3.0g total fat
(1.7g saturated fat); 849kJ (203 cal);
32.6g carbohydrate; 9.6g protein; 2.3g fibre

1 medium mango (430g), peeled, chopped coarsely
1 cup (250ml) buttermilk
⅓ cup (95g) skim-milk fruit-flavoured yogurt
2 tablespoons lime juice

1  Blend ingredients until smooth.

### Sarah's diary
*Trying to cut out my
morning coffee on the way
to work is proving to be a
challenge – I had no idea
how reliant I was on the
caffeine to wake me up.
Thankfully, the mango lassi
was lovely. The sandwich
was nice; I cooked my own
beef because I'm not a fan
of the deli-bought beef
slices. Dinner was very
filling – the weather was
still balmy when I got
home, so I cooked my fish
on the bbq. Could've killed
for a gin & tonic to wash it
all down with, though.*

### Pamela's diary
*More tastings today, which
involved chocolate: I did
taste the tiniest amounts
possible, though. More
confessions – I broke the
weigh-yourself-once-a-week
rule this morning, based on
the feeling that my skirt felt
slightly less snug than
usual, and, to my delight,
I have lost 0.6kg in just
two days, despite the glass
of wine and the tastings.
I know daily weight can
see-saw between one and
two kilos, but I just know
I've lost weight.*

Make sure the mango
you use is properly ripe,
and, if you like, use all
buttermilk and forget
about the yogurt.

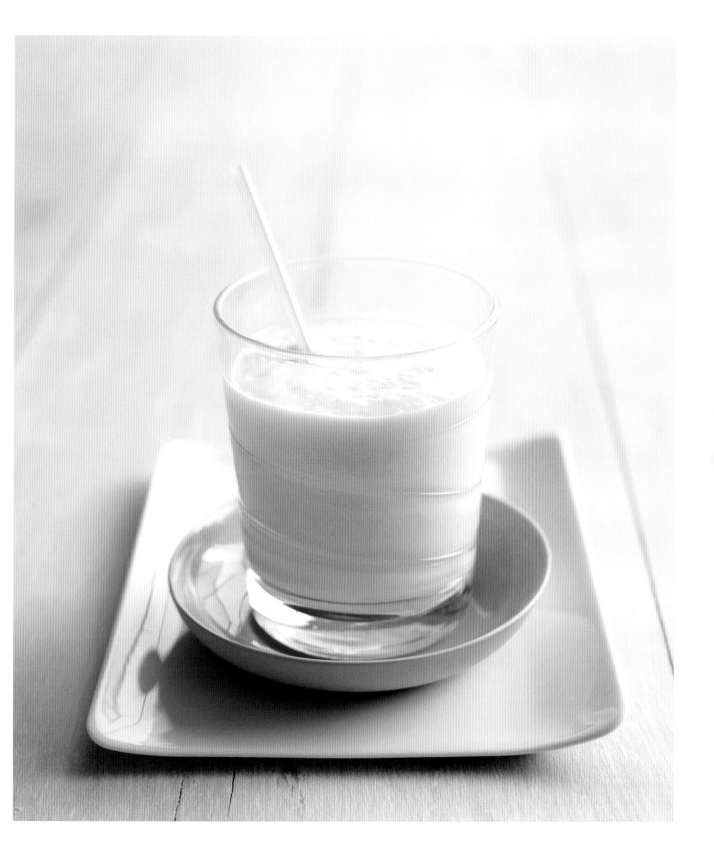

Use whatever cabbage you like; try the chinese variety (wombok), it's easy to shred finely. You can buy the roast beef, already cooked, from any deli.
Make the coleslaw the night before, then make the sandwich at lunch time the next day.

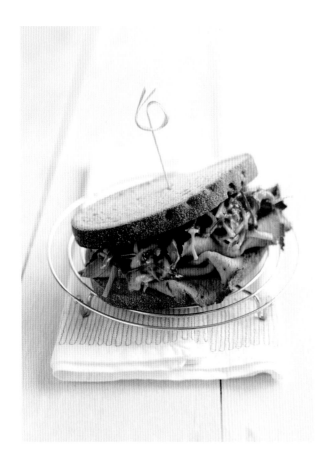

LUNCH

# roast beef and coleslaw on rye

**preparation time** 10 minutes **serves** 2
**nutritional count per serving** 9.8g total fat (2.6g saturated fat); 1731kJ (415cal); 51.1g carbohydrate; 25.0g protein; 9.7g fibre

1 cup (80g) finely shredded cabbage
1 small carrot (70g), grated coarsely
2 green onions, chopped finely
¼ cup (75g) 97% fat-free mayonnaise
1 tablespoon lemon juice
4 slices rare roast beef (120g)
4 slices rye bread (180g)

1  Combine cabbage, carrot, onion, mayonnaise and juice in medium bowl.
2  Divide beef between two slices of bread; top with coleslaw, then remaining bread.

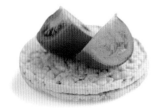

snack 2 corn thins with ½ small sliced tomato

Use any firm fish that's in season, it's cheaper that way. Sumac is a type of Middle-Eastern spice, now available from supermarkets. The flavour is slightly tart. If you can't find the spice, cook the fish without it.

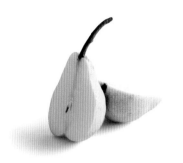

snack 1 small pear

# sumac fish with couscous salad

cooking-oil spray
1 small red onion (100g), chopped finely
1 clove garlic, crushed
2 small green zucchinis (180g),
    sliced diagonally
125g cherry or grape tomatoes
¼ cup coarsely chopped fresh mint
½ cup (125ml) vegetable stock
½ cup (100g) couscous
320g firm white fish fillets
2 teaspoons sumac
1 lemon

1  Spray medium frying pan with cooking oil; cook onion and garlic over heat, stirring, 1 minute. Add zucchini and tomatoes; cook, stirring occasionally, about 10 minutes or until vegetables soften. Remove from heat; stir in mint.
2  Bring stock to a boil in small saucepan; remove from heat, stir in couscous, stand 5 minutes. Stir into zucchini mixture.
3  Meanwhile, preheat grill. Sprinkle fish with sumac; grill until cooked, turning once.
4  Serve couscous topped with fish and lemon wedges.

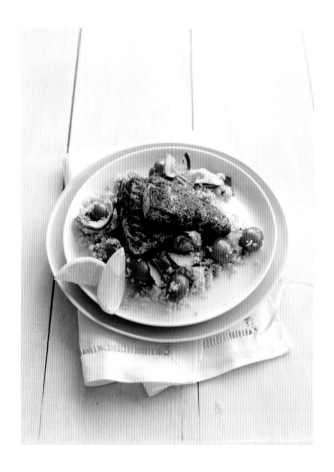

preparation time 10 minutes
cooking time 20 minutes  serves 2
nutritional count per serving  5.6g total fat
(1.4g saturated fat); 1739kJ (416 cal);
45.4g carbohydrate; 42.4g protein; 5.2g fibre

# Day 4 Menu

bran and cranberry muesli | orange-roasted kumara and tuna salad | warm tandoori chicken salad

# bran and cranberry muesli

**preparation time** 5 minutes  **serves** 2
**nutritional count per serving**  1.7g total fat
(0.4g saturated fat); 606kJ (145cal);
24.0g carbohydrate; 6.0g protein; 4.5g fibre

1 cup (90g) rolled oats
¾ cup (55g) All-Bran
¼ cup (35g) dried cranberries
⅔ cup (160ml) skim milk
½ cup (75g) fresh blueberries

1  Combine oats, bran and cranberries in small bowl to make muesli mixture.
2  Place ⅓ cup muesli in each bowl; top with milk and berries.
Store remaining muesli in an airtight container for Day 12 and Day 20.

### Sarah's diary
*First taste of All Bran in my life this morning – I have always steered well clear of it, but it's actually not that bad. I couldn't get any fresh blueberries, so used thawed frozen berries instead. We had so many tastings in the Kitchen today; I held a teaspoon in my hand to taste, rather than the usual dessertspoon! Prepared lunch last night, was quick and easy, and tasted great today. Met friends after work for drinks, and settled for a mineral water rather than a riesling – a healthier, and a far cheaper, option.*

### Pamela's diary
*Feeling good, not hungry; even went for a brisk walk this morning. Breakfast and lunch were great, but we weren't happy with the tandoori chicken for dinner: we've had a play with the recipe, you'll love it now. Last night, just to be sociable, I ate an olive and a dolmades, and was overcome by the oiliness; last week I would have scoffed at least six olives, and who knows how many dolmades. It really doesn't take the body long to start cleaning up its act.*

If you don't want to use dried cranberries, use sultanas or raisins instead.

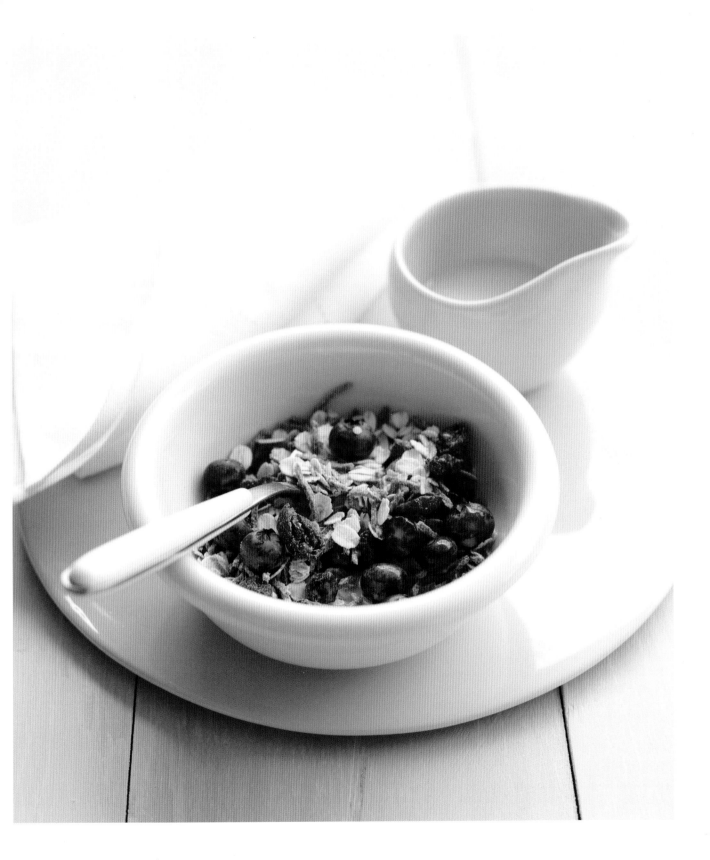

This recipe makes enough for 6 servings. If you don't feel like making some of the breakfasts we suggest, you can always have this muesli instead; remember, it's a ⅓ cup serving. You can always make a larger batch and keep it in an airtight container in the fridge.

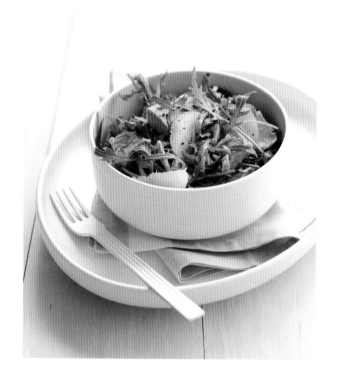

Substitute any type of pumpkin for the kumara, if you like. It's best to prepare the ingredients the night before, then make the salad in the morning for lunch.

LUNCH

# orange-roasted kumara and tuna salad

**preparation time** 10 minutes (plus cooling time)
**cooking time** 20 minutes  **serves** 2
**nutritional count per serving**  2.6g total fat
(0.8g saturated fat); 1195kJ (286 cal);
37.0g carbohydrate; 25.1g protein; 6.2g fibre

1 medium kumara (400g), peeled, cut into 2cm pieces
2 teaspoons finely grated orange rind
185g can tuna in springwater, drained, flaked
80g baby rocket leaves
1 large orange (300g), peeled, segmented
2 tablespoons orange juice
1 tablespoon light soy sauce
½ small red onion (50g), sliced thinly

1  Preheat oven to 180°C/160°C fan-forced.
2  Place kumara on oven tray; sprinkle with rind.
Roast, uncovered, about 20 minutes; cool.
3  Combine kumara with remaining ingredients
in medium bowl.

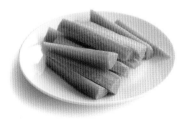

snack 1 small carrot

Chicken tenderloins are available from chicken shops and most supermarkets. If you like, you can use the same weight of lean chicken breast fillet and cut the fillet into long thin strips for quick cooking.

DINNER

# warm tandoori chicken salad

⅓ cup (95g) skim-milk natural yogurt
⅓ cup coarsely chopped fresh coriander
2 tablespoons lemon juice
6 small pappadums (20g)
280g chicken tenderloins
2 tablespoons tandoori powder
cooking-oil spray
100g baby spinach leaves
1 lebanese cucumber (130g), halved lengthways,
   sliced thickly
125g yellow teardrop tomatoes

1  Combine yogurt, coriander and juice in small bowl.
2  Cook pappadums in microwave oven on MEDIUM (50%) for about 40 seconds; break into pieces.
3  Sprinkle chicken with tandoori powder; spray with cooking oil. Cook chicken on heated grill plate (or grill or barbecue). Slice thickly.
4  Combine spinach, cucumber and tomatoes in medium bowl; add chicken. Serve salad sprinkled with pappadums, then drizzled with coriander yogurt.

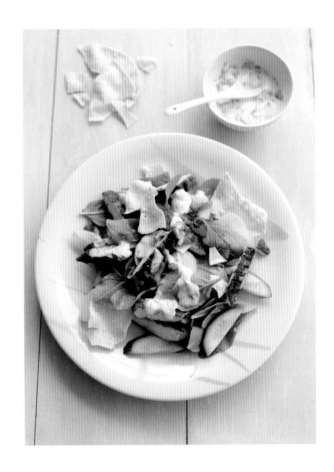

preparation time 15 minutes
cooking time 10 minutes serves 2
nutritional count per serving 4.8g total fat
(1.0g saturated fat); 1053kJ (252 cal);
10.7g carbohydrate; 38.7g protein; 4.4g fibre

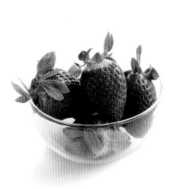

snack 125g strawberries

# Day 5 Menu

tomato and egg muffin | ricotta, basil and ham wrap | sesame beef stir-fry

# tomato and egg muffin

**preparation time** 5 minutes
**cooking time** 5 minutes  **serves** 2
**nutritional count per serving** 7.3g total fat
(1.9g saturated fat); 953kJ (228 cal);
24.2g carbohydrate; 14.5g protein; 3.9g fibre

cooking-oil spray
2 eggs
2 multigrain english muffins, split
1 small tomato (90g), sliced thinly
2 teaspoons balsamic vinegar

1  Spray medium frying pan with cooking oil. Fry eggs until cooked as you like.
2  Meanwhile, toast muffins.
3  Divide tomato between two muffin halves; sprinkle with vinegar, top with eggs, then remaining muffin halves.

## Sarah's diary

*Arrived at work to find bags upon bags of lollies for the kids' party cake book we're working on. Usually, I would have nose-dived into the pile of sugar, but I just kept on walking. Breakfast was yum; kept me going all morning. Ate my lunch in the local park, then went for a stroll to get my legs moving…they say that every bit counts! Stir-fry for dinner took next to no time to make, which was great after a long day at work. I think my boyfriend is quite envious of all this delicious food I'm eating – perhaps he'll join me!*

## Pamela's diary

*Happy with the egg and tomato muffin for breakfast and loved the wrap at lunch time. The stir-fry for dinner was spot-on – it is my favourite meal so far, with just the right balance of flavours and chilli heat, and, I'm sure if you cooked this for people not on a diet, they wouldn't know the difference. More chocolate testing today, and we've started work on another party cake book, the Test Kitchen is littered with lollies – that tests us.*

You can cut out another gram of fat by poaching the eggs in gently simmering water.

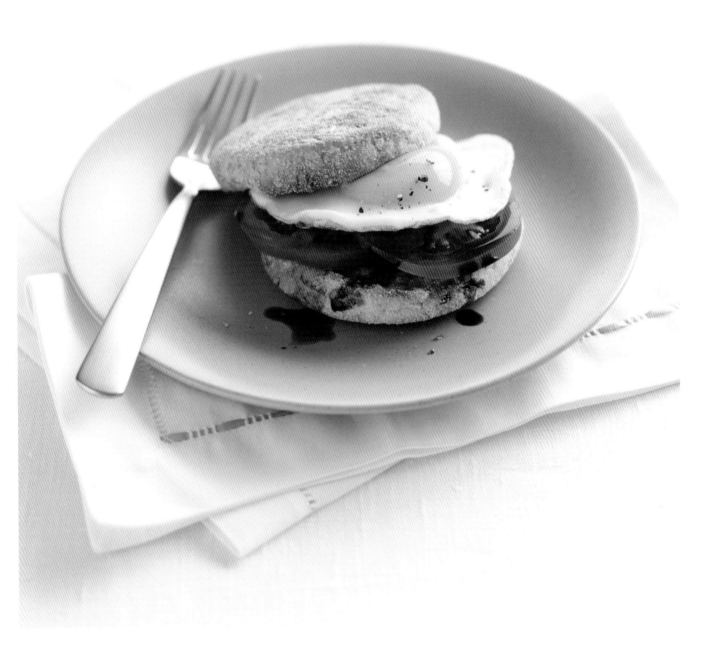

# ricotta, basil and ham wrap

**preparation time** 5 minutes
**cooking time** 3 minutes  **serves** 2
**nutritional count per serving**  4.7g total fat
(2.3g saturated fat); 886kJ (212 cal);
24.1g carbohydrate; 16.1g protein; 3.7g fibre

2 small zucchini (180g)
¼ cup (60g) low-fat ricotta cheese
3 rye mountain bread wraps (90g)
75g shaved ham
¼ cup coarsely chopped fresh basil

1  Preheat sandwich press.
2  Slice zucchini lengthways into ribbons using a
vegetable peeler.
3  Divide cheese among wraps; top with zucchini,
ham and basil. Roll to enclose.
4  Toast wraps in sandwich press for about 3 minutes;
cut in half to serve.

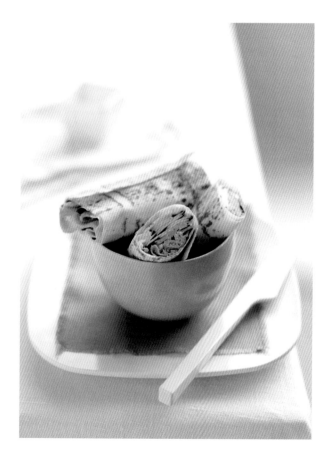

It's not vital to "toast" the wrap
in a sandwich press, but it
does give it a bit of a crisp
texture. Make the wrap in the
morning ready for lunch.

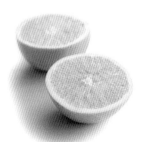

snack 1 medium orange

# sesame beef stir-fry

½ cup (100g) couscous
½ cup (125ml) boiling water
2 teaspoons sesame seeds
180g rump steak, sliced thinly
1 small red onion (100g), cut into wedges
1 clove garlic, crushed
1 baby buk choy (150g), quartered
1 fresh long red chilli, sliced thinly
2 tablespoons beef stock
2 tablespoons oyster sauce
2 tablespoons light soy sauce
150g snow peas, sliced thinly

1  Combine couscous with the water in medium heatproof bowl, cover; stand 5 minutes.
2  Meanwhile, toast sesame seeds in heated wok about 30 seconds; transfer to small bowl.
3  Stir-fry beef in heated wok until browned; transfer to another small bowl.
4  Stir-fry onion in heated wok 1 minute. Add garlic, buk choy and chilli; stir-fry 1 minute. Add stock, sauces and beef; stir-fry until hot. Remove from heat; stir in peas.
5  Serve couscous topped with stir-fry and sprinkled with sesame seeds.

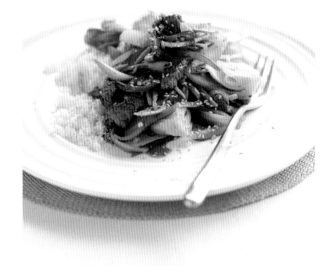

**preparation time** 10 minutes
(plus standing time)
**cooking time** 10 minutes  **serves** 2
**nutritional count per serving**  5.6g total fat
(2.1g saturated fat); 1643kJ (393 cal);
51.3g carbohydrate; 31.3g protein; 4.1g fibre

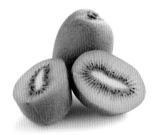

snack 2 apricots, plums
or kiwifruit

# Day 6 Menu

corn fritters | asparagus frittata with rocket | linguine marinara

# corn fritters

**preparation time** 10 minutes
**cooking time** 10 minutes **serves** 2
**nutritional count per serving** 6.1g total fat
(1.4g saturated fat); 1476kJ (353 cal);
50.4g carbohydrate; 19.3g protein; 8.4g fibre

1 egg
310g can corn kernels, rinsed, drained
½ small red onion (50g), sliced thinly
½ cup (80g) wholemeal self-raising flour
⅓ cup (80ml) skim milk
cooking-oil spray
⅓ cup (65g) low-fat cottage cheese

1  Whisk egg in medium bowl; stir in corn, onion, flour and milk.
2  Spray large frying pan with cooking oil. Pour ⅓-cup of batter into heated pan; cook about 2 minutes or until bubbles appear. Turn fritters; cook until lightly browned on the other side.
3  Serve warm fritters dolloped with cheese; sprinkle with fresh dill or parsley, if you like.

## Sarah's diary

My usual Saturday morning breakfast at the café downstairs was canned this morning, made the corn fritters instead and was not disappointed. Still managed to read the newspapers and have a peppermint tea at the café in the afternoon. Lunch was good; I loved the asparagus. Had invited friends over for dinner, so I just doubled the recipe for the marinara – everyone was thrilled that they too were eating a low-fat feast. I joined in for a glass of wine, but stopped after one.

## Pamela's diary

I shared the corn fritters with my two granddaughters this morning – very well-received by all. Loved the frittata, but marinara is not my favourite thing in life. I love seafood, but prefer it unadorned. My local seafood shop usually does a really outstanding marinara mix, but this week it missed the mark for me; mind you, I ate the lot. If you like, you could use just prawns instead of the mix.

40

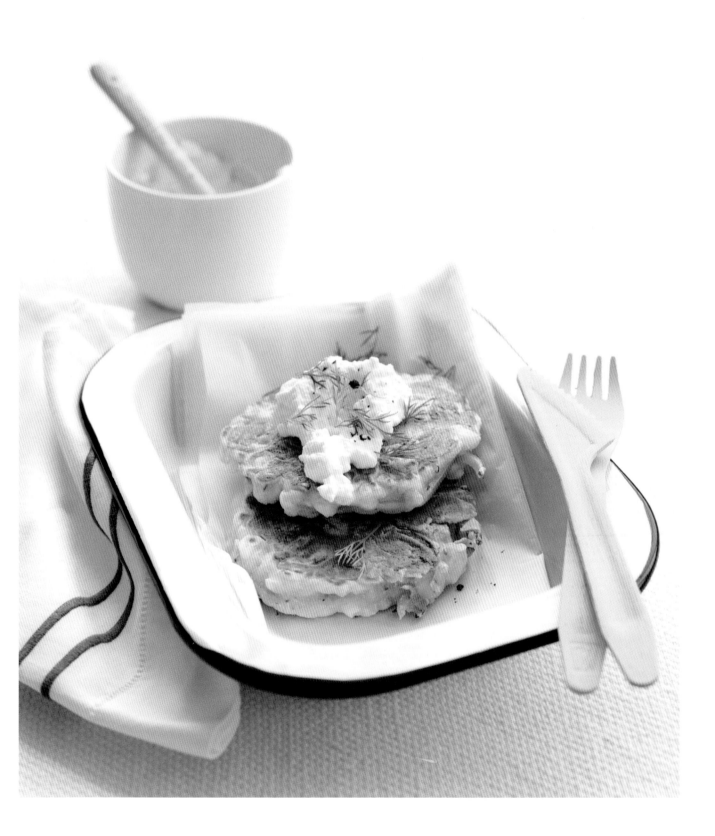

If you'd rather cook fresh corn, the easiest way is to coat the cob lightly with cooking oil spray, then cook it over the barbecue or on a griddle pan, turning the cob until it's lightly charred all over. Then, place the cob on a board and slice off the kernels.

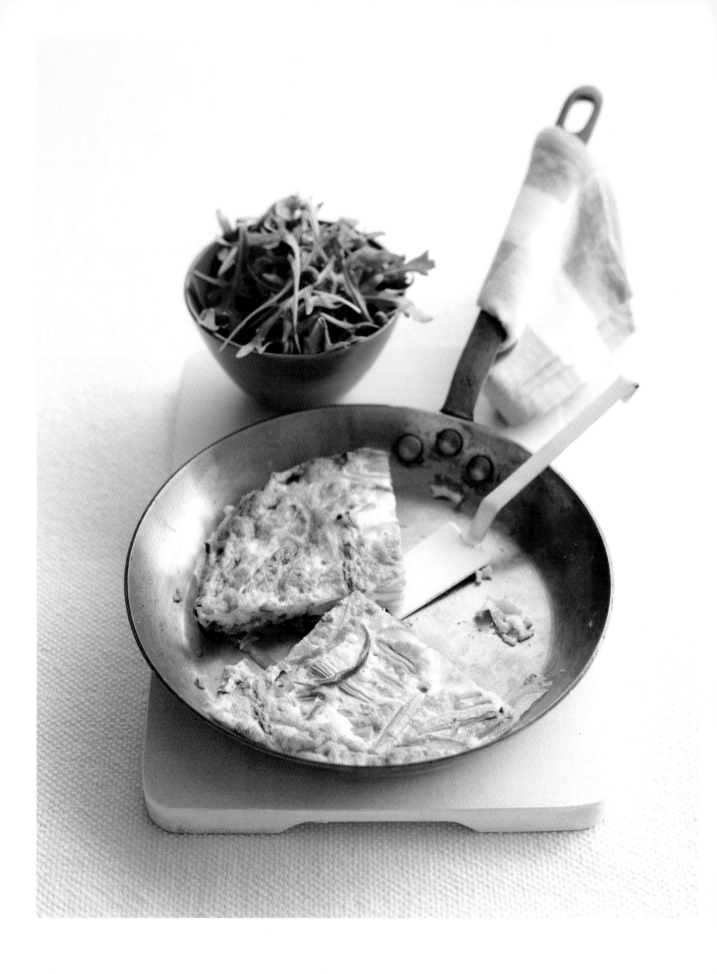

If the handle of your frying pan is not heatproof, cover it with aluminium foil before placing it under the grill.

Frittata is delicious served warm, but if you like it cold, and want to take it to work, make it the evening before, keep it in the fridge, then wrap it in plastic the next morning.

LUNCH

# asparagus frittata with rocket

**preparation time** 10 minutes
**cooking time** 15 minutes  **serves** 2
**nutritional count per serving**  6.3g total fat
(1.8g saturated fat); 614kJ (147 cal);
5.4g carbohydrate; 16.3g protein; 1.9g fibre

cooking-oil spray
1 small red onion (100g), sliced thinly
170g asparagus, trimmed, cut into 2cm lengths
2 eggs
2 egg whites
2 tablespoons low-fat cottage cheese
40g baby rocket leaves
2 tablespoons lemon juice
2 teaspoons drained baby capers, rinsed

1  Preheat grill.
2  Spray small frying pan with cooking oil; cook onion over heat, stirring, 1 minute. Add asparagus; cook, stirring, 2 minutes.
3  Meanwhile, combine eggs, egg whites and cheese in a medium jug. Pour over asparagus mixture in pan. Cook, uncovered, about 5 minutes or until frittata is browned underneath.
4  Place pan under grill for about 5 minutes or until frittata is set.
5  Combine remaining ingredients in medium bowl; serve frittata with salad.

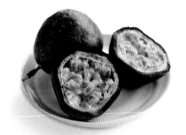

snack 2 passionfruit

This is a really simple recipe. There's only one thing to be careful of – don't overcook the seafood – if you do, it will be tough and leathery.

Use any pasta shape you like – and don't overcook it either. Cooked pasta with a little bit of bite left in it is better for your digestive system.

# linguine marinara

**preparation time** 5 minutes
**cooking time** 15 minutes  **serves** 2
**nutritional count per serving**  7.2g total fat
(1.8g saturated fat); 2387kJ (571 cal);
61.9g carbohydrate; 60.1g protein; 6.4g fibre

150g linguine pasta
400g marinara mix
1 small brown onion (80g), chopped finely
2 cloves garlic, crushed
1 fresh small red thai chilli, chopped finely
400g can diced tomatoes
⅓ cup coarsely chopped fresh flat-leaf parsley

1  Cook pasta in large saucepan of boiling water until tender; drain.
2  Meanwhile, cook marinara mix in heated large frying pan, stirring, for 2 minutes; drain.
3  Add onion, garlic and chilli to same heated pan; cook, stirring, about 5 minutes or until onion softens. Add undrained tomatoes; cook, 5 minutes. Return seafood to pan; cook, stirring occasionally,  for about 2 minutes. Stir in parsley.
4  Serve pasta with marinara sauce.

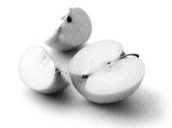

snack 1 small apple

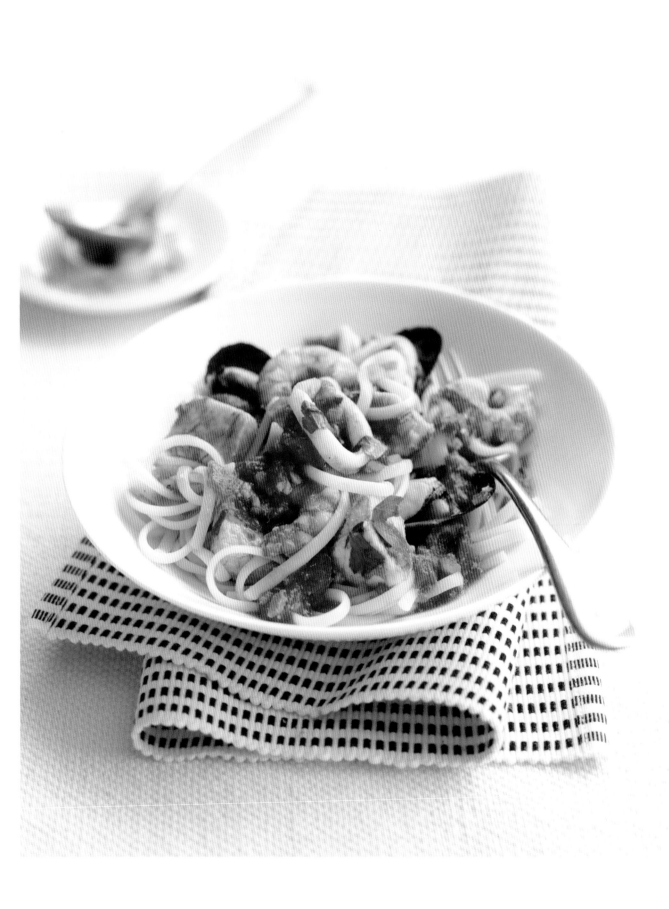

# Day 7 Menu

date loaves | warm roasted vegie salad | pork cutlets with chickpea puree

# date loaves

**preparation time** 10 minutes
**cooking time** 20 minutes  **serves** 2
**nutritional count per serving**  6.5g total fat
(1.3g saturated fat); 1183kJ (283 cal);
46.4g carbohydrate; 8.2g protein; 2.2g fibre

**cooking-oil spray**
**1 egg white**
**2 teaspoons vegetable oil**
**½ cup (75g) self-raising flour**
**⅓ cup (80ml) skim milk**
**1 tablespoon finely chopped dried dates**
**1 tablespoon brown sugar**
**1 tablespoon low-fat ricotta cheese**

**1**  Preheat oven to 180°C/160°C fan-forced. Spray two holes of ½-cup (125ml) rectangular or round muffin pan with cooking oil.
**2**  Whisk egg white with a fork in medium bowl; stir in oil, flour, milk, dates and sugar, do not overmix. Divide mixture between pan holes.
**3**  Bake about 20 minutes. Serve warm loaves with cheese.

## Sarah's diary
*Dragged boyfriend out of bed bright and early to go for a walk to the beach. Even though there were complaints about "being up too early for a Sunday", I think he secretly enjoyed the fresh air. Got home and made the date loaves – such a great breakfast. Went with friends for a picnic at lunchtime, so I just packed up my vegie salad and took it with me. After one week of this diet, I'm feeling great; I probably look the same, but I feel a lot healthier.*

## Pamela's diary
*Those date loaves are just divine, especially eaten warm. If I could be trusted not to eat them at random, I'd make quite a lot and freeze them, they would thaw really well in a microwave oven – I guess they'd take up to a minute to reheat. I've always been a fan of roasted vegie salads, but with lashings of olive oil; I love them hot, warm or cold.*

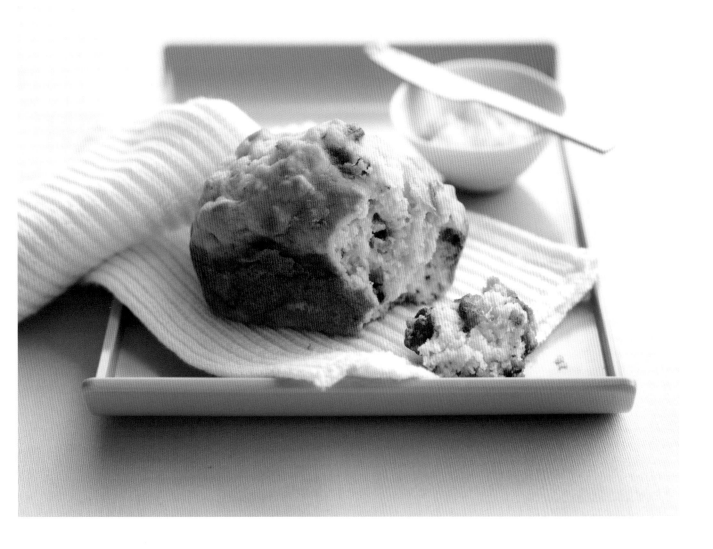

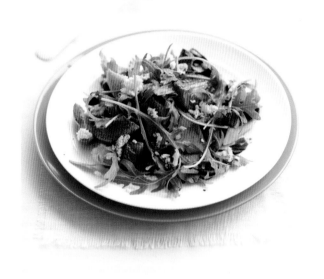

Instead of roasting the vegies, you can char-grill them on a barbecue or a grill pan for a more smoky flavour.
The salad can be made a day ahead, then warmed through in a microwave oven. Add the cheese last.

LUNCH

# warm roasted vegie salad

**preparation time** 10 minutes
**cooking time** 25 minutes  **serves** 2
**nutritional count per serving**  2.6g total fat
(1.2g saturated fat); 673kJ (161 cal);
20.8g carbohydrate; 10.0g protein; 7.0g fibre

2 flat mushrooms (160g), halved
1 small kumara (250g), cut into 4cm pieces
1 small red capsicum (150g), cut into 4cm pieces
2 small tomatoes (180g), quartered
2 cloves garlic, chopped coarsely
¼ cup coarsely chopped fresh flat-leaf parsley
50g baby rocket leaves
1 tablespoon balsamic vinegar
2 tablespoons low-fat ricotta cheese

1  Preheat oven to 220°C/200°C fan-forced.
2  Combine vegetables and garlic in large baking dish. Roast, uncovered, about 25 minutes.
3  Combine roasted vegetables with parsley, rocket and vinegar in large bowl.
4  Serve salad sprinkled with cheese.

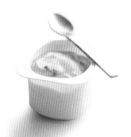

snack 100g skim-milk fruit-flavoured yogurt

preparation time 10 minutes
cooking time 10 minutes serves 2
nutritional count per serving 7.2g total fat
(1.7g saturated fat); 1225kJ (293 cal);
16.0g carbohydrate; 37.3g protein; 7.1g fibre

DINNER

# pork cutlets with chickpea puree

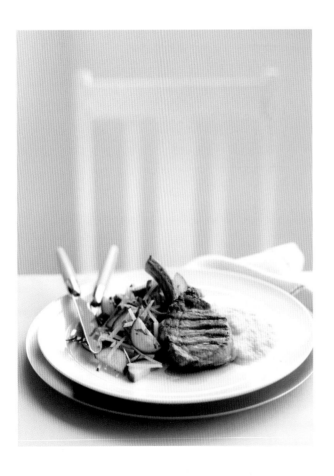

2 x 125g cans chickpeas, rinsed, drained
2 tablespoons lemon juice
2 cloves garlic, crushed
1 teaspoon ground fennel
⅓ cup (80ml) warm water
2 pork cutlets (470g), trimmed
cooking-oil spray
5 red radishes (300g), cut into matchsticks
1 lebanese cucumber (130g), chopped coarsely
⅓ cup coarsely chopped fresh flat-leaf parsley

1  Process chickpeas, juice, garlic and fennel until
combined. Add the water; process until smooth.
2  Spray pork with cooking oil; cook pork on heated
grill plate (or grill or barbecue).
3  Meanwhile, combine remaining ingredients in
medium bowl.
4  Serve pork with salad and chickpea puree.

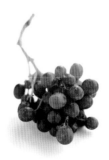

snack 125g grapes

# Day 8 Menu

berry smoothie | lentil, tuna and tomato salad | crunchy chicken salad cups

# berry smoothie

**preparation time** 5 minutes  **serves** 2
**nutritional count per serving**  0.5g total fat
(0.2g saturated fat); 711kJ (170 cal);
26.9g carbohydrate; 12.2g protein; 3.4g fibre

250g strawberries
½ cup (75g) fresh or frozen blueberries
1 cup (250ml) skim milk
¾ cup (200g) skim-milk fruit-flavoured yogurt

1  Blend ingredients until smooth.

### Sarah's diary
*Smoothie tasted good, ate
my snack at breakfast,
too as I felt a bit peckish.
Had more tastings for
the chocolate book we're
working on – Pamela and I
were very restrained (I think
everyone at work is starting
to believe that we're taking
this diet seriously!). None of
the food has tasted diet-like
yet: I'm surprised, because
there's so little fat in the
recipes. Ate dinner before
going to a work function,
which was a good move,
otherwise I would've eaten
all the beautiful canapés
they were serving.*

### Pamela's diary
*Clean, clean, clean is how
I feel, and just a little bit
smug and worthy; I'm
certainly not hungry, and
I'm certainly losing weight,
what more can a girl ask
for. Just over one third of
the way there and I've lost
two kilos, and am feeling
very well. Back to work
today, some kind person
even commented on my
weight loss.*

You decide on the berry
combination – they're all
really good for you. Match
the flavours with the yogurt.

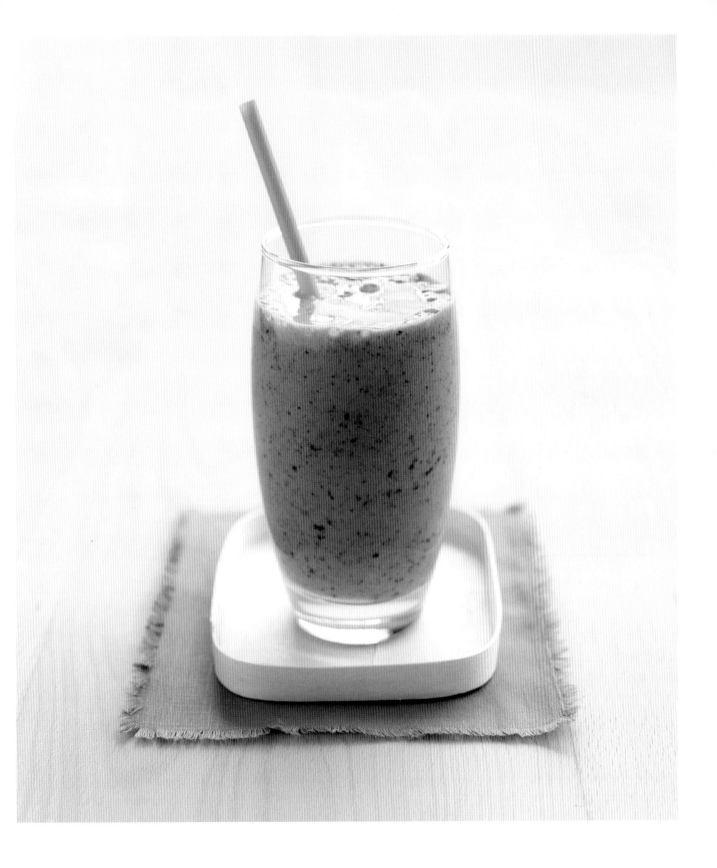

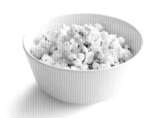

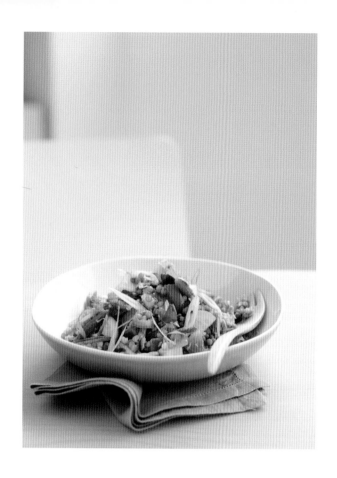

snack 2 cups plain popcorn
Popcorn is a great snack –
even without the butter. Put
2 tablespoons of popping corn
into a large saucepan, cover with
a tightly fitting lid. Turn the heat
to high and wait for the popping
to start. Turn off the heat and wait
for the popping to stop before
removing the lid. This will give
you 2 cups of popcorn.

LUNCH

# lentil, tuna and tomato salad

**preparation time** 10 minutes  **serves** 2
**nutritional count per serving**  2.7g total fat
(0.8g saturated fat); 911kJ (218 cal);
18.3g carbohydrate; 26.7g protein; 6.3g fibre

This is a perfectly portable
lunch. It can be made a
day ahead.

400g can brown lentils, rinsed, drained
185g can tuna in springwater, drained, flaked
1 lebanese cucumber (130g), chopped coarsely
2 small tomatoes (180g), chopped coarsely
2 green onions, sliced thinly
⅓ cup coarsely chopped fresh flat-leaf parsley
1 clove garlic, crushed
2 tablespoons lemon juice
¼ cup (45g) drained cornichons, halved

1  Combine ingredients in medium bowl.

**preparation time** 10 minutes (plus cooling time)
**cooking time** 10 minutes  **serves** 2
**nutritional count per serving** 4.5g total fat
(1.1g saturated fat); 895kJ (214 cal);
4.3g carbohydrate; 36.1g protein; 5.5g fibre

DINNER

# crunchy chicken salad cups

220g chicken breast fillet
cooking-oil spray
½ cup (100g) low-fat cottage cheese
3 trimmed celery stalks (300g), chopped coarsely
4 green onions, sliced thinly
2 teaspoons coarsely chopped fresh dill
1 clove garlic, crushed
6 small iceberg lettuce leaves

**1**  Spray chicken with cooking oil; cook chicken in heated small frying pan. Remove from heat; cool.
**2**  Shred chicken coarsely; combine in medium bowl with cheese, celery, onion, dill and garlic.
**3**  Divide chicken mixture among lettuce leaves.

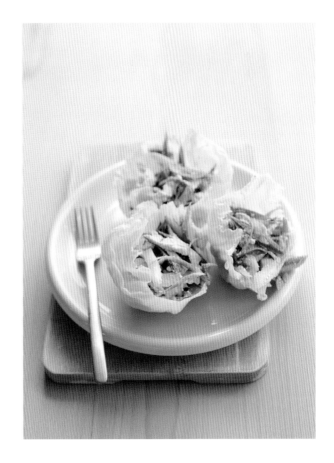

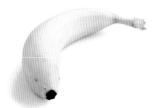

snack 1 small banana

# Day 9 Menu

spinach omelette | turkey and cranberry wrap | prosciutto-wrapped lamb with roasted kipflers

## spinach omelette

**preparation time** 5 minutes
**cooking time** 5 minutes  **serves** 2
**nutritional count per serving** 5.7g total fat
(1.6g saturated fat); 878kJ (210 cal);
21.2g carbohydrate; 16.3g protein; 4.0g fibre

1 egg
4 egg whites
2 green onions, chopped finely
cooking-oil spray
30g baby spinach leaves
2 tablespoons coarsely chopped fresh mint
2 slices rye bread (90g), toasted
1 tablespoon low-fat ricotta cheese

1  Whisk egg, egg whites and onion in small jug.
2  Spray small frying pan with cooking oil; heat pan. Pour egg mixture into pan; cook, tilting pan, until mixture is almost set. Sprinkle spinach and mint over half the omelette; fold omelette over to enclose filling, then cut in half.
3  Spread toast with cheese; serve with omelette.

### Sarah's diary
*Managed to get my belt in an extra notch this morning; the diet is obviously working! I have so much basil in the garden at the moment, I decided to throw a bit into the spinach omelette for breakfast. Such a great, fresh flavour. Lunch was yum – I can't remember the last time I had turkey and cranberry. Had a friend's birthday dinner, so had to miss the diet dinner. After scanning the menu at the Asian restaurant for a healthy option, I went for the steamed vegie dumplings – they certainly hit the spot.*

### Pamela's diary
*Sarah has the tiniest waist of anyone I've ever known, and it's getting tinier, she looks terrific. We both agree this diet is really good, easy to follow, well-balanced, with a wide variety of food and, for those of us watching the budget, and who isn't these days, it's quite inexpensive. We've deliberately avoided exotic ingredients, we bought everything we needed from mainstream supermarkets.*

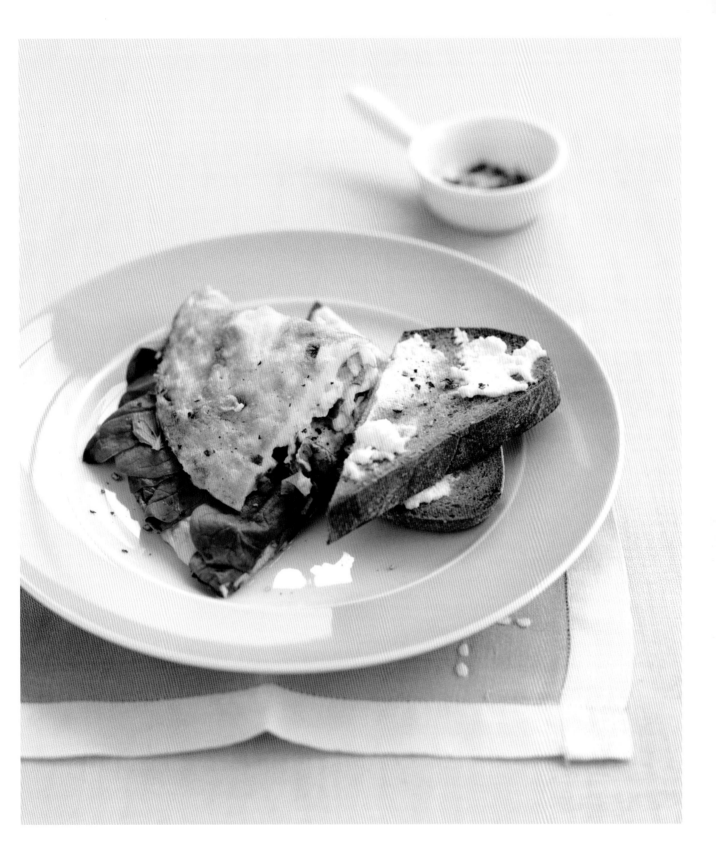

Save the egg yolks by freezing them in ice block trays and use for making something decadent after the diet. Don't be afraid to turn the heat up high when you're cooking the omelette; fast and hot is the way to go.

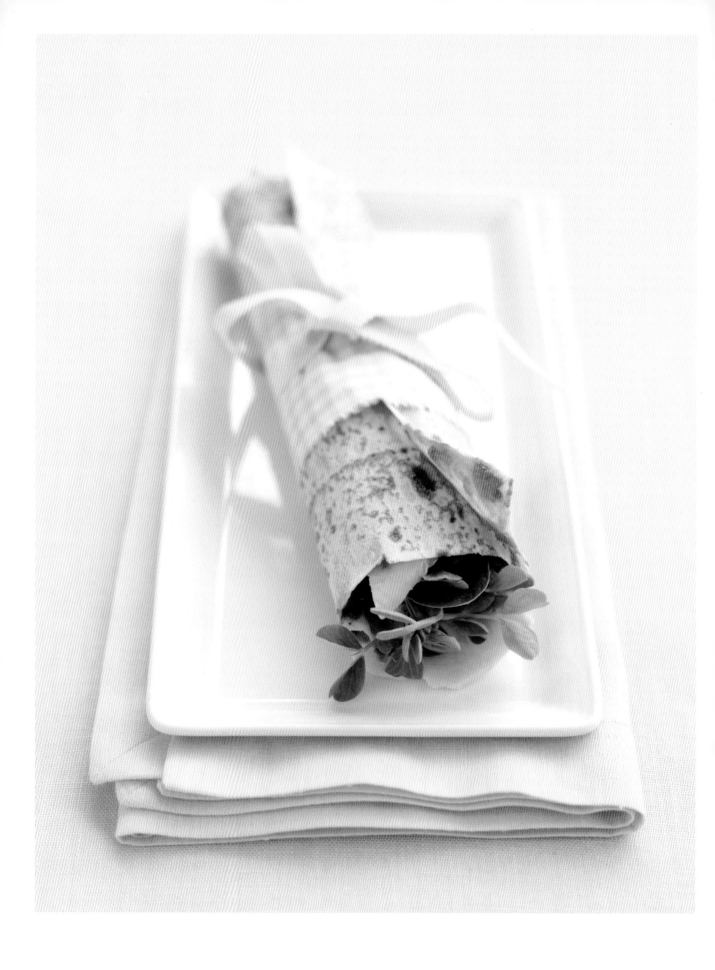

Snow pea sprouts are often hard to get. Substitute with regular bean sprouts or any other kind you like. By all means, use rocket, or any left-over greens instead of the spinach. These wraps travel well; make them the night before, if you like.

# turkey and cranberry wrap

**preparation time** 5 minutes  **serves** 2
**nutritional count per serving**  2.1g total fat
(0.4g saturated fat); 849kJ (203 cal);
27.6g carbohydrate; 16.7g protein; 2.5g fibre

2 rye mountain bread wraps (60g)
2 tablespoons cranberry sauce
80g shaved turkey
30g snow pea sprouts
30g baby spinach leaves

1  Spread wraps with sauce; top with remaining ingredients. Roll to enclose.

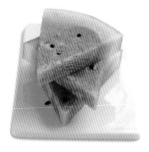

snack 200g watermelon

# prosciutto-wrapped lamb with roasted kipflers

**preparation time** 15 minutes
**cooking time** 30 minutes  **serves** 2
**nutritional count per serving**  7.3g total fat
(3.3g saturated fat); 1488kJ (356 cal);
33.7g carbohydrate; 34.8g protein; 7.3g fibre

The ruby red grapefruit is lovely in this recipe, but you could use orange segments. Don't bother to peel the potatoes, the skin is good for you.

400g kipfler potatoes, halved lengthways
200g lamb backstrap
1 clove garlic, sliced finely
2 slices prosciutto (30g)
150g green beans, trimmed
1 ruby red grapefruit (350g), segmented
¼ cup coarsely chopped fresh flat-leaf parsley
30g reduced-fat fetta cheese, crumbled

1  Preheat oven to 220°C/200°C fan-forced.
2  Place potato in small ovenproof dish; roast, uncovered, 15 minutes.
3  Meanwhile, cut small slits in lamb; fill each slit with a garlic slice. Wrap prosciutto around lamb. Cook lamb in heated medium frying pan, 1 minute each side. Remove from pan; place on top of potato.
4  Roast lamb and potato, uncovered, about 10 minutes.
5  Meanwhile, boil, steam or microwave beans until tender.
6  Combine beans with remaining ingredients in medium bowl.
7  Slice lamb, serve with potato and salad.

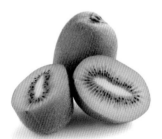

snack 2 kiwifruit

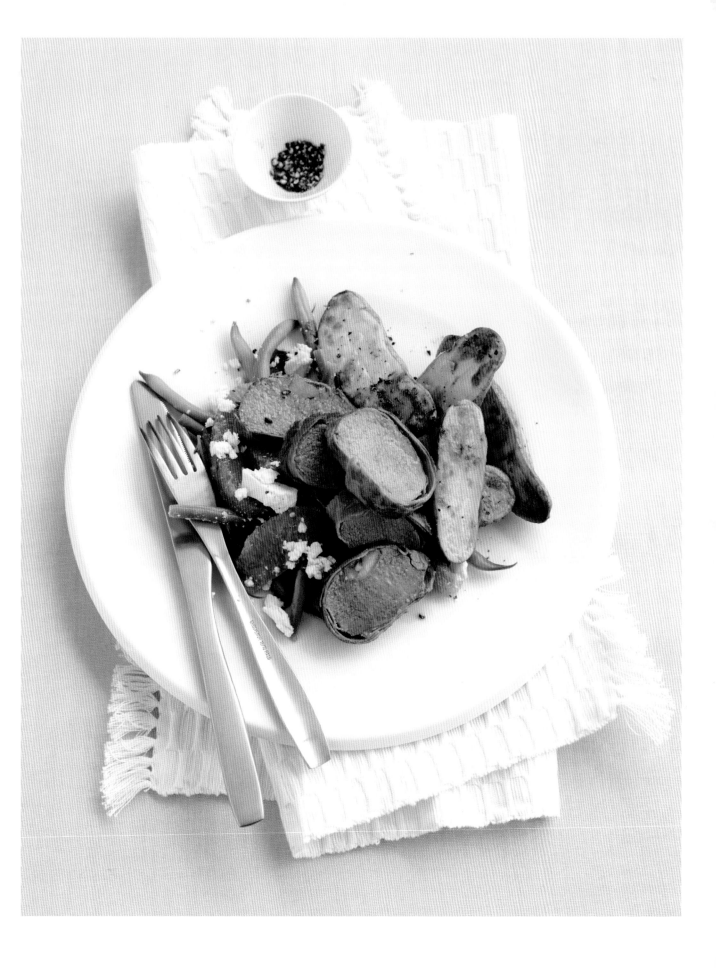

# Day 10 Menu

ricotta and banana on toast | beef, mint and cucumber salad | cumin fish with roasted corn salsa

# ricotta and banana on toast

**preparation time** 5 minutes  **serves** 2
**nutritional count per serving**  2.9g total fat
(1.3g saturated fat); 966kJ (231 cal);
40.6g carbohydrate; 7.7g protein; 5.0g fibre

2 tablespoons low-fat ricotta cheese
2 slices rye bread (90g), toasted
2 small bananas (260g), sliced thickly
1 teaspoon honey
pinch ground cinnamon

1  Divide cheese between slices of toast; top with banana, drizzle with honey, then sprinkle with cinnamon.

## Sarah's diary
*I've lost 2.3kg and I feel good. Breakfast felt like a real treat; I love banana and cinnamon. Pamela and I both enjoyed lunch – it was so filling. Shops had sold out of red capsicum, so I had to use cherry tomatoes in the salsa for dinner instead, and it worked just fine. The testing for the chocolate cookbook continued today… truffles galore – usually I would've devoured a whole tray, but I was very pleased with my restraint and only had a crumb.*

## Pamela's diary
*Felt a bit on the greedy side today; there seemed to be more food than on other days. When we first tested the recipes for this diet, we were tasting the meals for a whole day all at the one time, so we decided that there really was only one way to test the diet properly, and that was to do it over the full three weeks. We always knew that we would be interrupted by tastings for other cookbooks and various family functions, but we figured, that's life.*

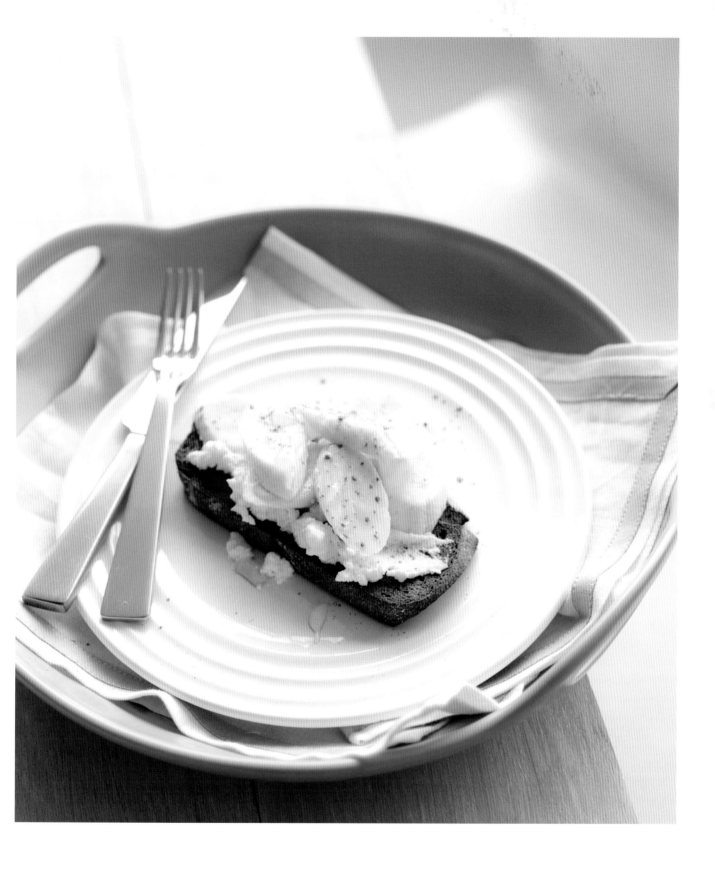

If you're taking this salad to work, hold the lemon juice until you're ready to eat. Otherwise, eat the salad while the beef is still warm.

LUNCH

# beef, mint and cucumber salad

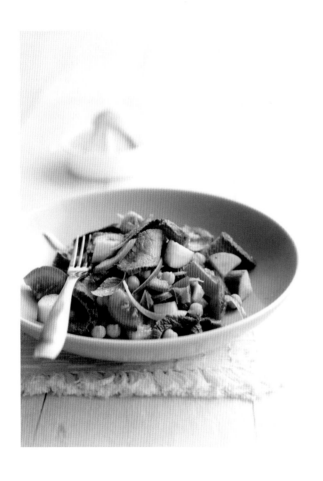

200g rump steak
cooking-oil spray
300g can chickpeas, rinsed, drained
1 lebanese cucumber (130g), chopped coarsely
2 small tomatoes (180g), chopped coarsely
½ small red onion (50g), sliced thinly
⅓ cup coarsely chopped fresh mint
¼ cup (60ml) lemon juice

1   Spray beef with cooking oil. Cook beef in heated small frying pan; remove from heat. Cover; stand 5 minutes.
2   Slice beef thinly; combine with remaining ingredients in medium bowl.

**preparation time** 10 minutes (plus standing time)
**cooking time** 5 minutes  **serves** 2
**nutritional count per serving**  6.0g total fat
(1.5g saturated fat); 1145kJ (274 cal);
19.2g carbohydrate; 31.7g protein; 7.5g fibre

snack 1 small red capsicum with 1 tablespoon low-fat cottage cheese

If limes are too expensive,
use lemons instead.
Any firm white fish is good
for this recipe.

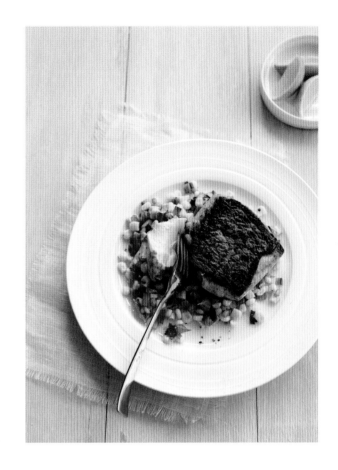

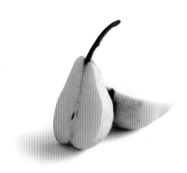

snack 1 small pear

DINNER

# cumin fish with roasted corn salsa

2 trimmed corn cobs (500g)
⅓ cup coarsely chopped fresh coriander
1 small red capsicum (150g), chopped finely
3 green onions, chopped finely
2 tablespoons lime juice
300g firm white fish fillets
1 teaspoon ground cumin

**preparation time** 10 minutes
**cooking time** 10 minutes  **serves** 2
**nutritional count per serving** 5.7g total fat
(1.2g saturated fat); 1534kJ (367 cal);
33.6g carbohydrate; 39.9g protein; 9.5g fibre

**1**  Cut kernels from corn cobs; roast corn in heated medium frying pan, stirring constantly. Transfer to medium bowl.
**2**  Stir in coriander, capsicum, onion and juice.
**3**  Sprinkle fish with cumin; cook in same heated pan.
**4**  Serve corn salsa topped with fish. Serve with lime wedges, if you like.

# Day 11 Menu

watermelon, raspberry and cranberry salad | chicken waldorf salad | beef rissoles with beetroot salad

# watermelon, raspberry and cranberry salad

**preparation time** 5 minutes **serves** 2
**nutritional count per serving** 0.9g total fat
(0.1g saturated fat); 757kJ (181 cal);
33.6g carbohydrate; 6.7g protein; 5.0g fibre

400g watermelon, cut into 2cm pieces
1 cup (135g) fresh raspberries
½ cup (125ml) diet cranberry juice
1 tablespoon coarsely chopped fresh mint
¾ cup (200g) skim-milk fruit-flavoured yogurt

1 Combine fruit, juice and mint in medium bowl. Serve topped with yogurt.

## Sarah's diary
*Went for a swim this morning; a refreshing way to start the day (and quite refreshing that my bikini fitted quite well!). I found breakfast quite light, but loved the watermelon and raspberries. Had tastings all morning for the Cooking from the Pantry cookbook – goodness me, the teaspoon I had of the chorizo & pumpkin risotto was so delicious, I could've eaten the entire bowl. Waldorf for lunch was nice; I didn't think the diet version would be good, but it surprised me. Dinner hit the spot; gotta love a rissole!*

## Pamela's diary
*Well, we're half way through now, and despite the interruptions, we're both liking this diet, and are even thinking of doing it again. We're both looking better, sleeping well, are more energetic and feeling good. The tastings in the Test Kitchen are a great temptation, but we have been restrained so far, although we both nearly "cracked" over a very good risotto today. I just read Sarah's diary entry – am glad I didn't have to beach-test a bikini.*

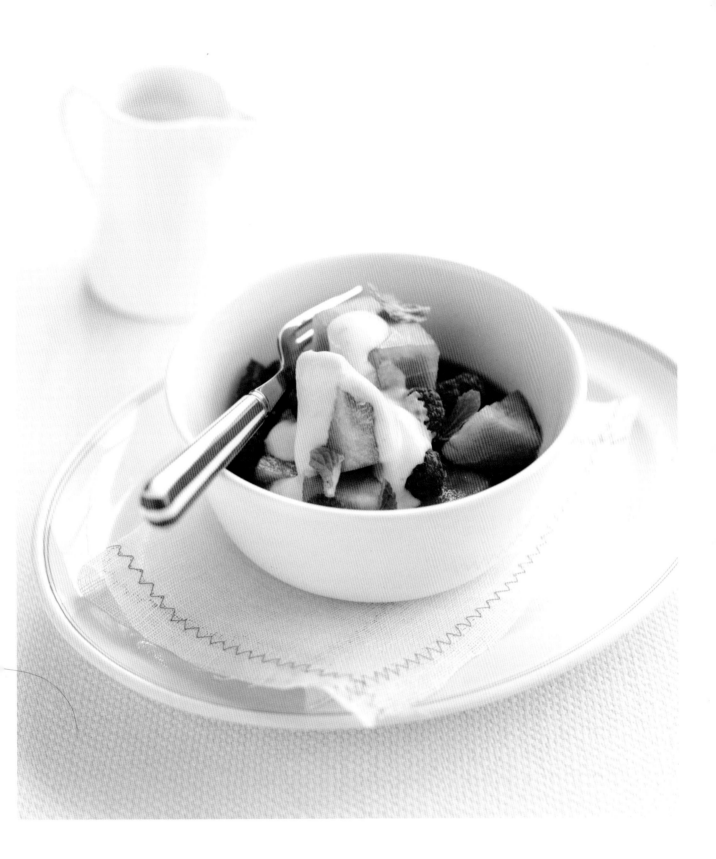

Strawberries are a good, and cheaper, substitute for raspberries. Match the yogurt flavour to your choice of berries.

**preparation time** 10 minutes (plus cooling time)
**cooking time** 10 minutes  **serves** 2
**nutritional count per serving**  2.7g total fat
(0.6g saturated fat); 761kJ (182 cal);
11.0g carbohydrate; 26.1g protein; 4.1g fibre

If you're taking this salad to work, make sure the apple is coated with the dressing to stop the flesh discolouring.

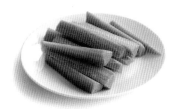

snack 1 small carrot

LUNCH

# chicken waldorf salad

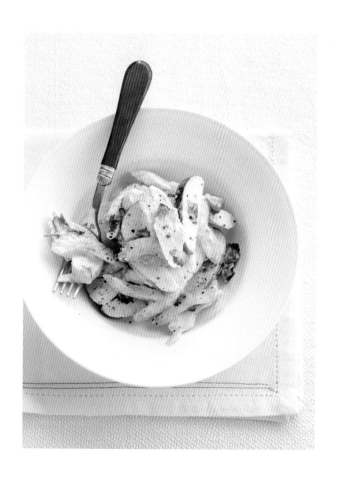

2 cups (500ml) water
200g chicken breast fillet
¼ cup (70g) skim-milk natural yogurt
2 tablespoons lemon juice
1 teaspoon wholegrain mustard
1 small red apple (130g), sliced thinly
3 trimmed celery stalks (300g), sliced diagonally
2 tablespoons coarsely chopped fresh flat-leaf parsley

1  Bring the water to the boil in a medium saucepan; add chicken. Simmer, covered, about 10 minutes or until chicken is cooked. Cool chicken in poaching liquid for 10 minutes; drain, then slice thickly.
2  Meanwhile, combine yogurt, juice and mustard in medium bowl. Add apple, celery, parsley and chicken; mix gently.

# beef rissoles with beetroot salad

220g lean beef mince
1 clove garlic, crushed
2 teaspoons ground cumin
cooking-oil spray
½ x 425g can baby beets, drained, halved
⅓ cup coarsely chopped fresh flat-leaf parsley
3 green onions, sliced thinly
1 tablespoon balsamic vinegar
2 tablespoons low-fat cottage cheese

**1** Combine beef, garlic and cumin in small bowl; shape mixture into four patties.
**2** Spray medium frying pan with cooking oil; heat pan. Cook patties in pan.
**3** Meanwhile, combine beetroot, parsley, onion and vinegar in medium bowl.
**4** Serve salad topped with patties and dolloped with cheese.

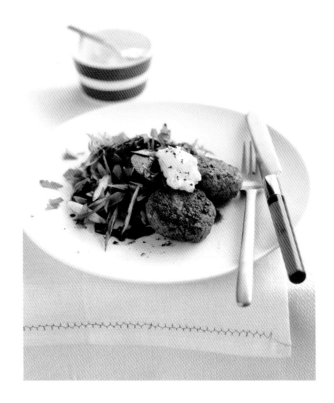

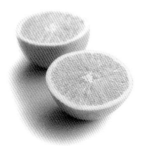

snack 1 medium orange

**preparation time** 10 minutes
**cooking time** 10 minutes  **serves** 2
**nutritional count per serving**  8.9g total fat
(3.4g saturated fat); 949kJ (227 cal);
7.9g carbohydrate; 27.1g protein; 2.9g fibre

# Day 12 Menu

muesli with pear and yogurt | egg and chive sandwich | ham, tomato and rocket pizza

## muesli with pear and yogurt

**preparation time** 5 minutes  **serves** 2
**nutritional count per serving**  1.8g total fat
(0.4g saturated fat); 896kJ (213 cal);
37.6g carbohydrate; 8.1g protein; 5.8g fibre

⅔ cup bran and cranberry muesli (see recipe, page 32)
1 small pear (180g), sliced thinly
½ cup (140g) skim-milk fruit-flavoured yogurt
⅓ cup (80ml) skim milk

1  Serve muesli topped with pear, then yogurt and milk.

### Sarah's diary
*Over half-way through and I'm really starting to notice the difference in how my clothes fit. Breakfast was quick to prepare and tasted great. We have a tradition in the Test Kitchen of having curried egg sandwiches once a fortnight for lunch, so today Pamela and I had our version of the egg sandwich, sans whole-egg mayo. I baby-sat the kids next door this evening, so we made the pizzas together – they were none the wiser that it was a lot healthier than the usual takeaway pizza.*

### Pamela's diary
*We have this Test Kitchen thing for curried egg sandwiches; Sarah rallied with her own very acceptable version, it has the yum factor without the fat. I'm not much of a pizza fan, but I have to say the pizza tonight was very good, and as for that muesli, I love it – the trick is to not eat too much of it.  If you're in a rush, or not into cooking breakfasts, especially during the week, remember, you can have this muesli for breakfast every day if you like.*

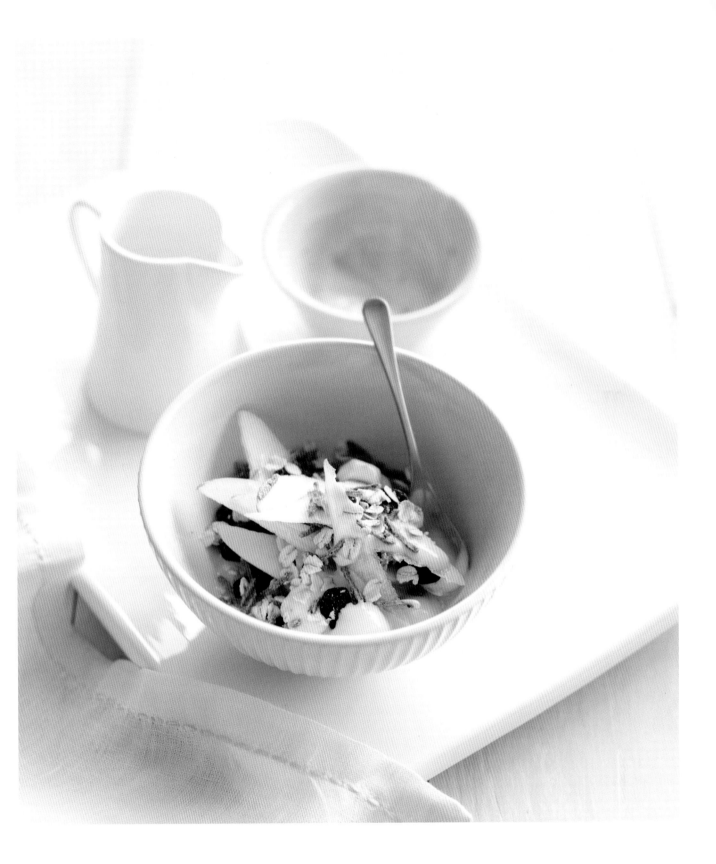

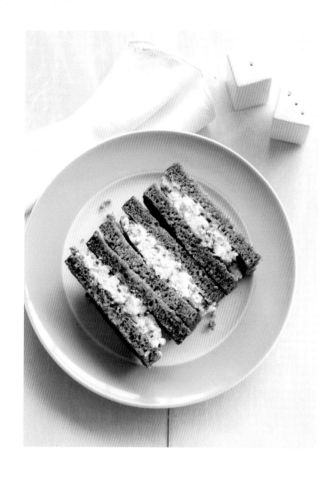

This is the perfect portable lunch. Boil the eggs the night before and make the filling and the sandwiches in the morning. Wrap them well in plastic wrap. If you like, add in some curry powder to taste.

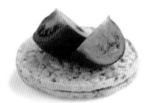

snack 2 corn thins with ½ small sliced tomato

LUNCH

# egg and chive sandwich

**preparation time** 5 minutes **serves** 2
**nutritional count per serving**  8.5g total fat (2.6g saturated fat); 1375kJ (329 cal); 40.6g carbohydrate; 19.2g protein; 6.2g fibre

2 hard-boiled eggs, halved
1 tablespoons low-fat ricotta cheese
2 tablespoons low-fat cottage cheese
2 tablespoons finely chopped fresh chives
4 slices rye bread (180g)

1  Place egg, cheeses and chives in medium bowl; using potato masher or back of fork, crush until combined.
2  Divide egg mixture between two slices of bread; top with remaining bread.

preparation time 10 minutes
cooking time 10 minutes  serves 2
nutritional count per serving  8.0g total fat
(3.5g saturated fat); 1559kJ (373 cal);
43.3g carbohydrate; 27.1g protein; 8.4g fibre

DINNER

# ham, tomato and rocket pizza

2 large wholemeal pitta bread (160g)
2 tablespoons tomato paste
150g shaved ham
250g cherry tomatoes, halved
¼ small red onion (25g), sliced thinly
⅓ cup (80g) low-fat ricotta cheese
30g baby rocket leaves
2 tablespoons finely shredded fresh basil

1  Preheat oven to 200°C/180°C fan-forced.
2  Place bread on oven trays; spread with paste. Divide ham, tomato and onion between bread; top with dollops of cheese.
3  Bake about 10 minutes. Serve sprinkled with rocket and basil.

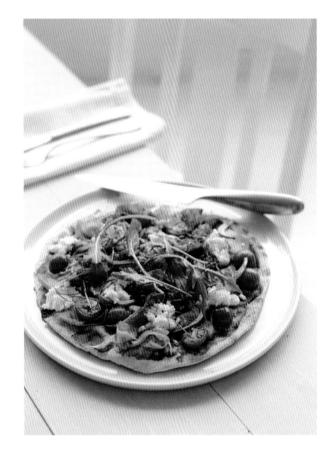

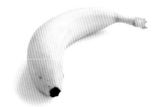

snack 1 small banana

# Day 13 Menu

roasted mushrooms with ricotta | chicken and pumpkin curry | hoisin pork with watercress salad

# roasted mushrooms with ricotta

**preparation time** 5 minutes
**cooking time** 15 minutes **serves** 2
**nutritional count per serving** 5.8g total fat
(3.4g saturated fat); 50.2kJ (120 cal);
2.4g carbohydrate; 12.4g protein; 4.7g fibre

4 flat mushrooms (320g)
½ cup (120g) low-fat ricotta cheese
2 tablespoons coarsely chopped fresh flat-leaf parsley
2 green onions, chopped finely
1 clove garlic, crushed

1  Preheat oven to 200°C/180°C fan-forced.
2  Place mushrooms, stem-side up, on oven tray.
Roast, uncovered, about 15 minutes.
3  Meanwhile, combine remaining ingredients in small bowl.
4  Serve mushrooms topped with cheese mixture.

## Sarah's diary

*Determined not to break the discipline on the weekend, my boyfriend and I had breakfast at home before going out for a coffee and newspaper read-a-thon. No complaints about the mushrooms – very filling. We had lunch quite late, but the curry didn't take long at all to make, and was satisfying. Met friends at the beach for late afternoon drinks; I settled for a small glass of wine. Had a friend's birthday bash at 8pm, so ate dinner just before I left home, which stopped me from tucking into the hummus!*

## Pamela's diary

*It's so easy to be slack on the weekends with diets, but we are both so inspired by this diet that we're determined to follow it as best we can. By now you'll have noticed that you eat quite a lot of dairy products in this diet, all low-fat, of course, and tomatoes feature quite a lot also. We've been quite strict about following the Dietary Guidelines for Australian Adults, with the correct balance of fruit, vegies, protein, dairy foods and carbs, etc.*

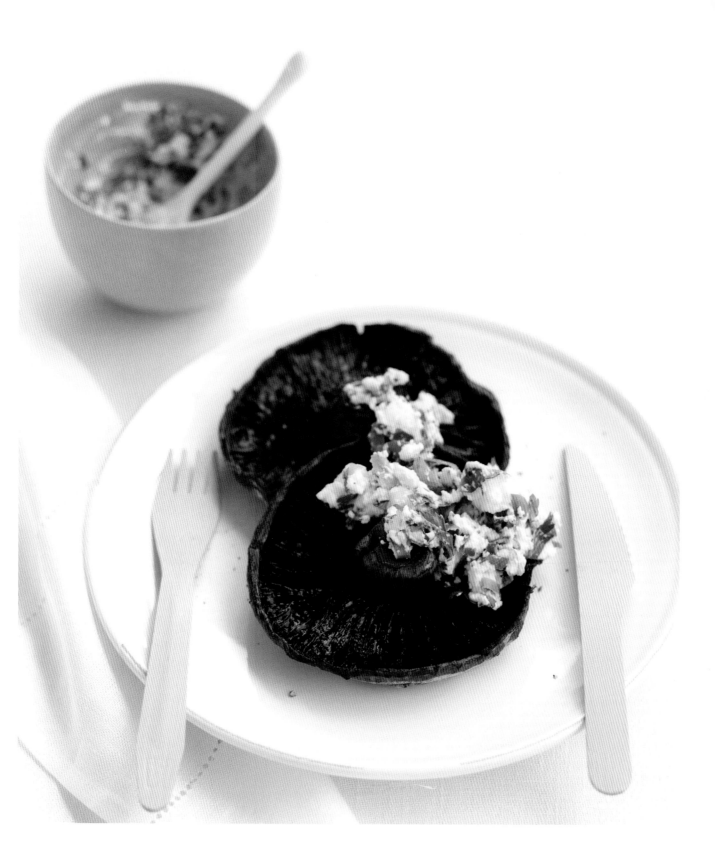

Try these mushrooms cooked on a
barbecue, they make a great breakfast for
lots of people – let your friends dollop their
own cheese mix onto the mushrooms.

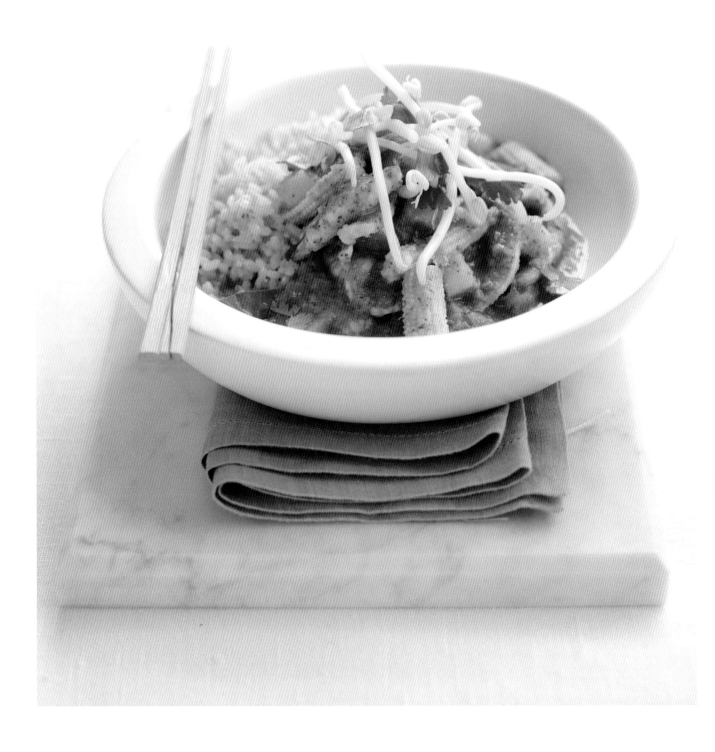

Brown rice takes about 30 minutes to cook, sometimes less depending on how crunchy you like it.
If you want takeaway curry, the whole recipe can be made a day ahead, then reheated in a microwave oven at lunch time.

# chicken and pumpkin curry

**preparation time** 15 minutes
**cooking time** 30 minutes  **serves** 2
**nutritional count per serving** 8.7g total fat
(4.6g saturated fat); 1973kJ (472 cal);
60.8g carbohydrate; 32.7g protein; 8.3g fibre

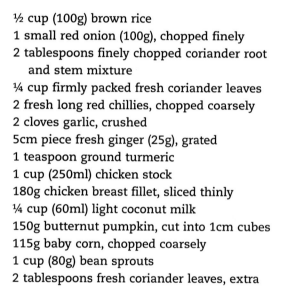

½ cup (100g) brown rice
1 small red onion (100g), chopped finely
2 tablespoons finely chopped coriander root
   and stem mixture
¼ cup firmly packed fresh coriander leaves
2 fresh long red chillies, chopped coarsely
2 cloves garlic, crushed
5cm piece fresh ginger (25g), grated
1 teaspoon ground turmeric
1 cup (250ml) chicken stock
180g chicken breast fillet, sliced thinly
¼ cup (60ml) light coconut milk
150g butternut pumpkin, cut into 1cm cubes
115g baby corn, chopped coarsely
1 cup (80g) bean sprouts
2 tablespoons fresh coriander leaves, extra

1  Cook rice in large saucepan of boiling water until tender; drain.
2  Meanwhile, blend onion, coriander root and stem mixture, coriander leaves, chilli, garlic, ginger and turmeric until smooth.
3  Cook paste in medium frying pan, stirring, until fragrant. Add stock, chicken and coconut milk; bring to a boil. Reduce heat; simmer, covered, 10 minutes.
4  Add pumpkin and corn to pan; simmer, uncovered, 10 minutes.
5  Serve rice topped with curry, sprouts and extra coriander.

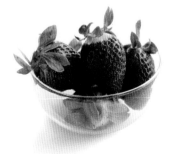

snack 125g strawberries

Watercress is a wonderful vegetable full of goodies like vitamins A, C and E, and is very high in iron and folic acid. It's a bit time-consuming to handle, as you need to pick off the sprigs, then wash and dry them carefully. We think it's worth the effort, but you can use spinach leaves instead, if you like.

DINNER

# hoisin pork with watercress salad

**preparation time** 15 minutes (plus standing time)
**cooking time** 10 minutes **serves** 2
**nutritional count per serving** 4.7g total fat
(1.2g saturated fat); 1066kJ (255 cal);
16.7g carbohydrate; 32.3g protein; 8.1g fibre

250g pork fillet
2 tablespoons hoisin sauce
cooking-oil spray
350g watercress, trimmed
⅓ cup coarsely chopped fresh mint
1 small green apple (130g), sliced thinly
½ small red onion (50g), sliced thinly
2 tablespoons lime juice
1 tablespoon light soy sauce
2cm piece fresh ginger (10g), grated
1 fresh small red thai chilli, chopped finely

**1** Spread pork with hoisin sauce. Spray medium frying pan with cooking oil; heat pan, cook pork. Cover pork; stand 5 minutes.
**2** Meanwhile, combine watercress, mint, apple and onion in medium bowl.
**3** Combine juice, soy sauce, ginger and chilli in small jug. Add to salad; toss to combine.
**4** Serve salad topped with sliced pork.

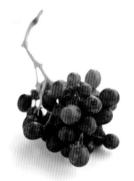

snack 125g grapes

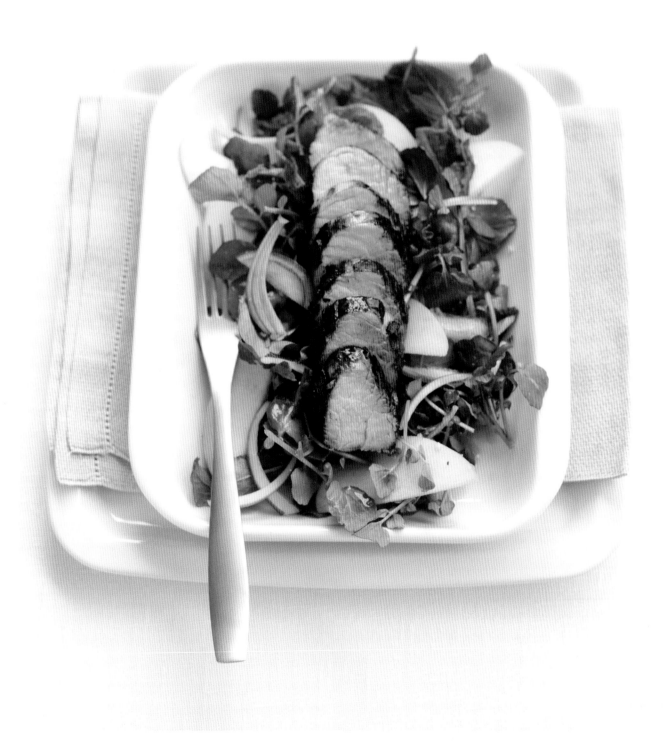

# Day 14 Menu

scrambled eggs with asparagus | thai-flavoured prawn salad | peppered beef with kumara wedges

# scrambled eggs with asparagus

**preparation time** 5 minutes
**cooking time** 10 minutes  **serves** 2
**nutritional count per serving**  6.4g total fat
(1.7g saturated fat); 518kJ (124 cal);
3.0g carbohydrate; 13.0g protein; 1.6g fibre

**170g asparagus, trimmed**
**cooking-oil spray**
**2 eggs**
**2 egg whites**
**2 tablespoons skim milk**
**1 small tomato (90g), chopped finely**
**2 tablespoons coarsely chopped fresh flat-leaf parsley**

1  Boil, steam or microwave asparagus until tender; drain
2  Meanwhile, spray medium frying pan with cooking oil. Whisk eggs, egg whites and milk in medium jug. Cook egg mixture in pan, over low heat, stirring, until almost set.
3  Serve asparagus and scrambled eggs sprinkled with tomato and parsley.

### Sarah's diary
*So nice to wake up this morning feeling good; had breakfast then did a bit of window shopping – saw a couple of things I'd like to try on after I finish the diet. Went to the seafood markets for lunch, so instead of the prawn salad, I had sushi. We had a barbecue on Sunday night, so I cooked my steak on the barbecue, too – I think everyone wanted to eat my kumara wedges, but I wasn't about to share. I didn't feel like the peppercorn sauce or broccolini with my steak, so just had a bit of rocket and tomato on the side, instead.*

### Pamela's diary
*Sunday was a bit of a disaster for me diet-wise; my family had a small gathering and, naturally enough for us, there was quite a lot of good food, good wine and fun involved. You could say I fell off the wagon, but there's always tomorrow and I've lost just over four kilos now. I wonder how long before Sunday's over-indulgences show up on the scales.*

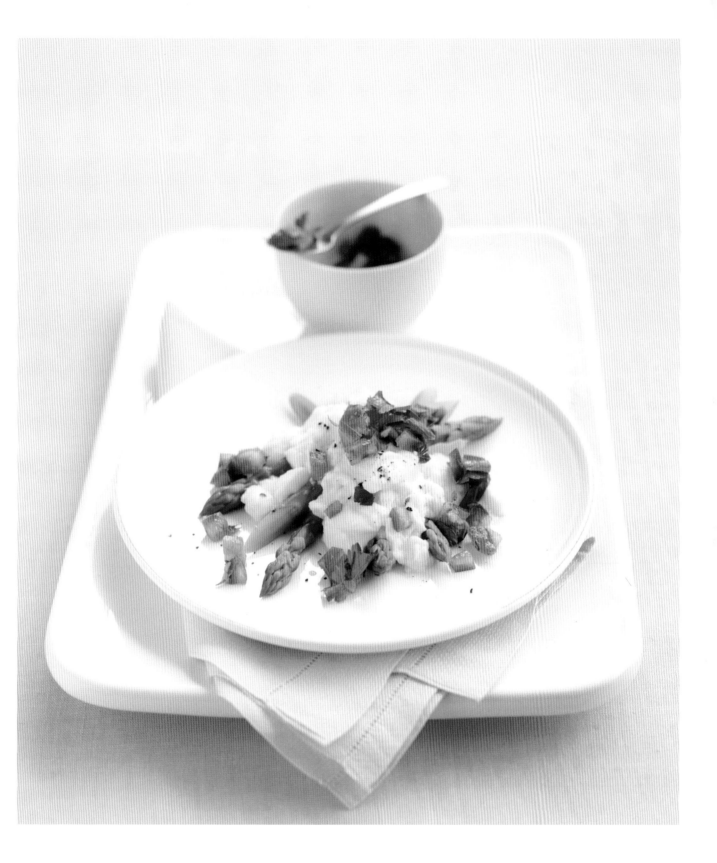

Scrambled eggs need to be cooked and stirred
gently until they are creamy and barely cooked.
Over-cooking will toughen them. Eat them
straight away or they'll become watery.

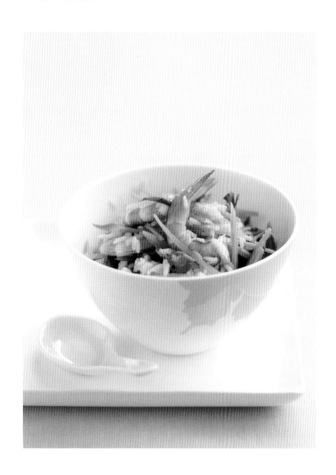

This is a perfect lunch to take to work: get all the ingredients ready the night before, then assemble the salad in the morning. It must be covered and refrigerated.

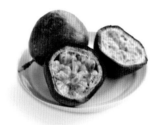

snack 2 passionfruit

# thai-flavoured prawn salad

**preparation time** 30 minutes (plus cooling time)
**cooking time** 25 minutes  **serves** 2
**nutritional count per serving**  2.3g total fat
(0.4g saturated fat); 1492kJ (357 cal);
61.1g carbohydrate; 19.5g protein; 4.6g fibre

¾ cup (150g) brown rice
250g cooked small prawns, shelled, deveined
1 small carrot (70g), grated coarsely
3 green onions, chopped finely
2 tablespoons coarsely chopped fresh coriander
1 clove garlic, crushed
1 teaspoon finely grated lime rind
¼ cup (60ml) lime juice
1 fresh small red thai chilli, chopped finely

1  Cook rice in large saucepan of boiling water, uncovered, until tender; drain, cool.
2  Combine rice in large bowl with remaining ingredients.

**preparation time** 5 minutes
**cooking time** 25 minutes  **serves** 2
**nutritional count per serving**  7.0g total fat
(2.5g saturated fat); 1367kJ (327 cal);
26.7g carbohydrate; 35.4g protein; 6.7g fibre

If you don't like green peppercorns, leave them out, and just season the steak with freshly ground black pepper.

DINNER

# peppered beef with kumara wedges

1 medium kumara (400g), cut into wedges
175g broccolini
2 beef eye-fillet steaks (250g)
cooking-oil spray
1 tablespoon drained green peppercorns
1 tablespoon buttermilk
½ cup (125ml) beef stock

1  Preheat oven to 200°C/180°C fan-forced.
2  Roast kumara on oven tray, uncovered, about 25 minutes.
Boil, steam or microwave broccolini until tender.
3  Meanwhile, spray beef with cooking oil; cook beef in
heated medium frying pan. Remove from heat;
cover with foil.
4  Add peppercorns, buttermilk and stock to pan; heat
without boiling.
5  Serve vegetables topped with beef, then drizzled with
peppercorn sauce.

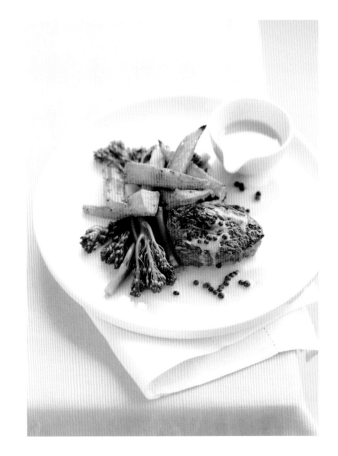

snack 100g skim-milk
fruit-flavoured yogurt

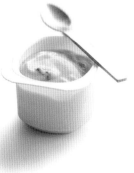

# Day 15 Menu

citrus salad | tuna, celery and dill sandwich | grilled mustard-chicken with potato smash

## citrus salad

**preparation time** 15 minutes  **serves** 2
**nutritional count per serving**  0.7g total fat
(0.1g saturated fat); 911kJ (218 cal);
40.6g carbohydrate; 8.9g protein; 5.4g fibre

**1 medium pink grapefruit (425g), segmented**
**2 medium navel oranges (480g), segmented**
**1 lime, segmented**
**60g strawberries, quartered**
**½ cup (125ml) unsweetened apple juice**
**¾ cup (200g) skim-milk fruit-flavoured yogurt**

**1**  Combine fruit and juice in medium bowl. Serve topped with yogurt.

### Sarah's diary
*I remember when we were really young, Mum always gave us grapefruit with our breakfast, but we would only eat it after it had been covered in about 10 spoons of sugar. Those days have gone, because I thoroughly enjoyed my fruit salad without any added sugar. Was starving by lunchtime and the sandwich hit the spot. Made my housemates dinner as well tonight – they claimed that it looked and tasted like "restaurant food". Well, if that's what they thought, then this diet can't be too bad!*

### Pamela's diary
*Fruit for breakfast is my favourite, it certainly is the lightest and cleanest food to start the day with, especially in the summer months. Mondays are usually a bit spartan in the Test Kitchen in terms of tastings, which is probably a good thing after yesterday, so, I'm back on the wagon and feeling happy about it. Loved the corn and potato smash for dinner.*

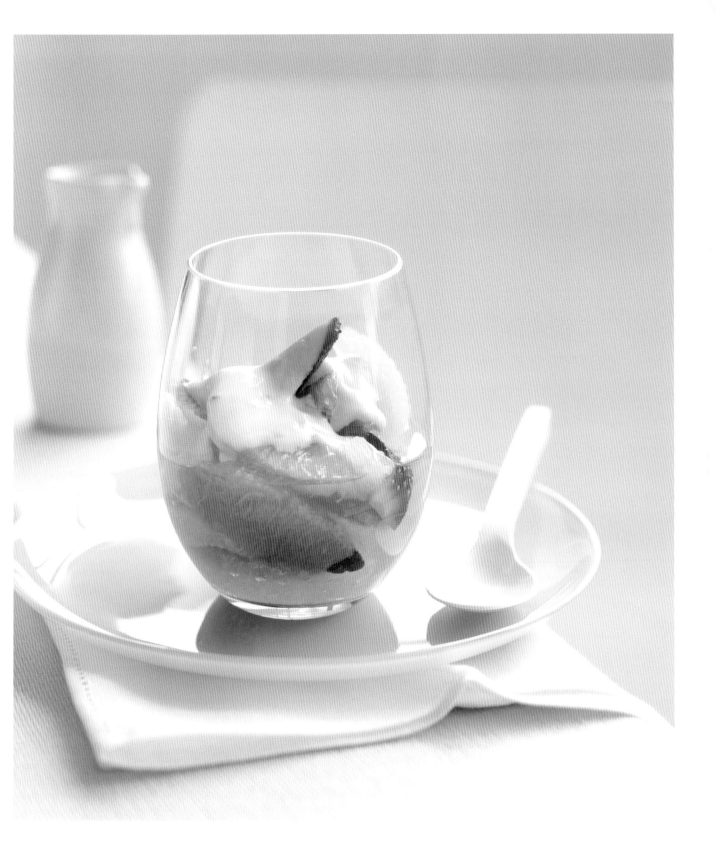

If you can't find pink (or ruby) grapefruit, use the ordinary grapefruit. Any combination of citrus fruit is fine; mix and match to suit your tastes.

# tuna, celery and dill sandwich

**preparation time** 10 minutes  **serves** 2
**nutritional count per serving**  6.0g total fat
(2.2g saturated fat); 1517kJ (363 cal);
42.5g carbohydrate; 29.9g protein; 8.4g fibre

185g can tuna in springwater, drained, flaked
2 trimmed celery stalks (200g), chopped finely
¼ small red onion (25g), chopped finely
2 tablespoons low-fat ricotta cheese
1 tablespoon coarsely chopped fresh dill
2 teaspoons rinsed, drained baby capers
4 slices rye bread (180g)
20g baby spinach leaves

1   Combine tuna, celery, onion, cheese, dill and capers
in medium bowl.
2   Divide spinach between two bread slices; top with
tuna mixture, then remaining bread.

If you're taking this
sandwich to work, make
the filling the night before,
then make the sandwich
in the morning. Put it in
the fridge when you arrive
at work. The spinach (or try
cos lettuce) will stop the
bread from turning soggy.

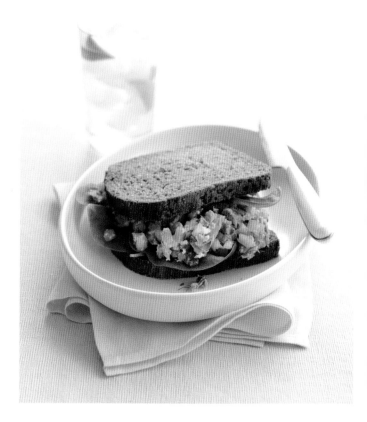

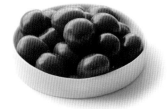

snack 125g grape tomatoes

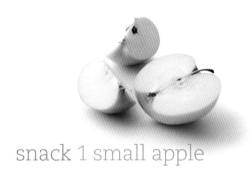

snack 1 small apple

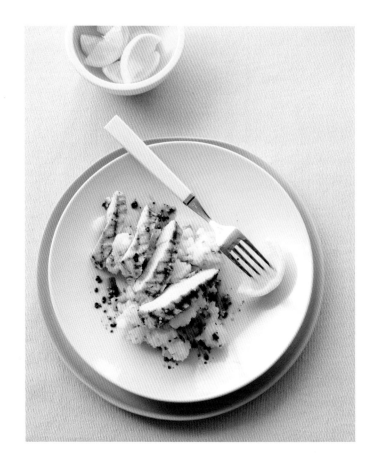

# grilled mustard-chicken with potato smash

**preparation time** 15 minutes
**cooking time** 15 minutes  **serves** 2
**nutritional count per serving**  5.7g total fat
(1.0g saturated fat); 2057kJ (492 cal);
62.6g carbohydrate; 41.3g protein; 10.8g fibre

3 medium potatoes (600g), unpeeled, halved
260g chicken breast fillet
cooking-oil spray
2 teaspoons wholegrain mustard
310g can corn kernels, rinsed, drained
2 tablespoons skim milk
2 tablespoons finely chopped fresh chives
1 lemon

1  Boil, steam or microwave potato until tender; drain.
2  Meanwhile, spray chicken with cooking oil; cook chicken on heated grill plate (or grill or barbecue), brushing occasionally with mustard. Cover chicken; stand 5 minutes, then slice thickly.
3  Combine potato, corn, milk and chives in large bowl; use potato masher or back of fork to crush mixture.
4  Serve chicken with potato smash and lemon wedges.

# Day 16 Menu

banana passionfruit smoothie | caesar salad | moussaka stack with lemon-yogurt dressing

# banana passionfruit smoothie

**preparation time** 5 minutes  **serves** 2
**nutritional count per serving**  0.5g total fat
(0.2g saturated fat); 1628kJ (246 cal);
46.0g carbohydrate; 12.2g protein; 2.9g fibre

**2 medium bananas (400g)**
**1 cup (250ml) skim milk**
**¾ cup (200g) skim-milk passionfruit-flavoured yogurt**
**Pinch ground nutmeg**

**1**  Blend bananas, milk and yogurt until smooth.
Serve smoothies lightly sprinked with nutmeg.

### Sarah's diary
*Nearly 3.5kg lost to date – I
really can't believe it. I
haven't felt this good in
a long time. My sugar
cravings have been well and
truly put to rest, finally! The
smoothie was good; I froze
my banana last night so I
had a super-icy breakfast.
The caesar salad was nice.
I'm not usually a big fan of
caesar salads but I actually
enjoyed this one. Dinner was
definitely my fave so far in
this whole diet…couldn't
believe it was diet food.*

### Pamela's diary
*Sarah looks wonderful; we
both agree this diet is the
best-ever, and let me tell you,
between us we've probably
tried every diet known to
mankind, so we know what
we're talking about. This
diet was originally devised
by home economist Amanda
Lennon, but Sarah and I
have tweaked the recipes
as we've been going along;
it's been very much a diet
in progress, so much so
that we've resolved to do
it again. What's to lose,
only more weight.*

We liked the flavour combination of passionfruit and banana, but any flavoured yogurt of your choice is fine. Bananas are at their sweetest when ripe, but slightly underripe bananas will make your digestive system work harder – so burning more kilojoules.

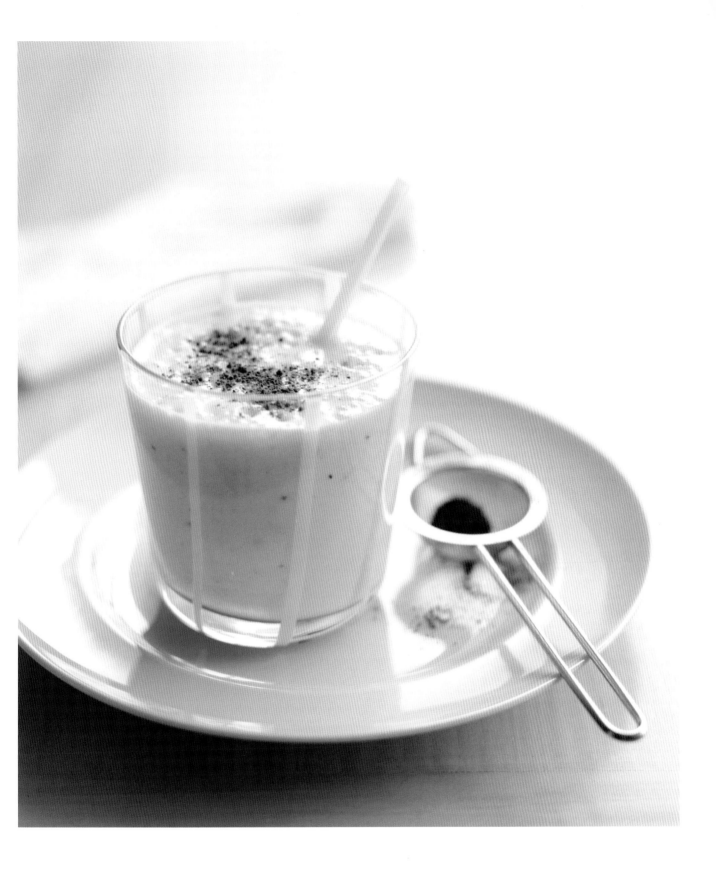

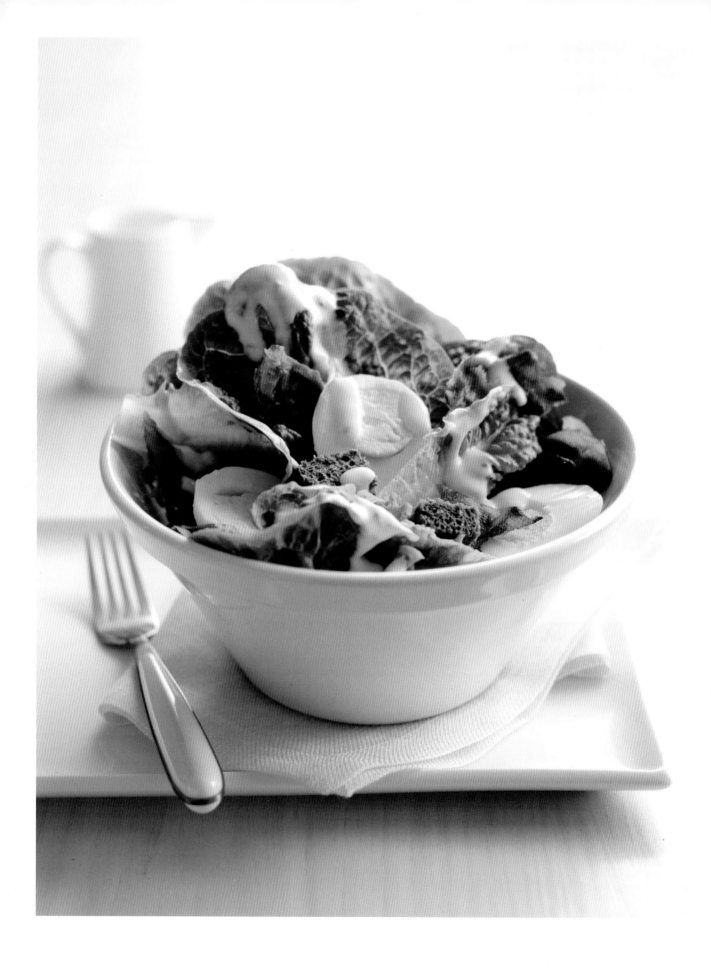

If you don't feel like toasting the bread cubes in the oven, toast the whole slices in the toaster or under a grill then cut the bread into small squares. Make sure you drain the anchovy fillet well between pieces of absorbent paper. If you want to have this delicious recipe at home, poach the egg instead of boiling it. Hold the yogurt dressing until you're ready to eat.

# caesar salad

**preparation time** 10 minutes
**cooking time** 5 minutes  **serves** 2
**nutritional count per serving** 5.6g total fat (1.4g saturated fat); 991kJ (237 cal); 25.7g carbohydrate; 17.1g protein; 6.9g fibre

2 slices rye bread (90g)
2 slices prosciutto (30g)
¼ cup (70g) skim-milk natural yogurt
1 tablespoon lemon juice
1 well-drained anchovy fillet, chopped finely
1 teaspoon dijon mustard
2 baby cos lettuces, trimmed, leaves separated
1 hard-boiled egg, sliced thinly

**1**  Preheat oven to 180°C/160°C fan-forced.
**2**  Remove crusts from bread; cut bread into small squares. Place on oven tray; toast about 5 minutes.
**3**  Meanwhile, cook prosciutto in medium heated frying pan until crisp; chop coarsely.
**4**  Combine yogurt, juice, anchovy and mustard in medium bowl. Add lettuce; toss to combine.
**5**  Serve lettuce mixture topped with toast, prosciutto and egg.

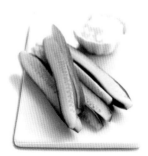

snack 1 lebanese cucumber with 1 tablespoon low-fat cottage cheese

# moussaka stack with lemon-yogurt dressing

**preparation time** 15 minutes
**cooking time** 15 minutes  **serves** 2
**nutritional count per serving** 6.9g total fat
(2.6g saturated fat); 957kJ (229 cal);
13.5g carbohydrate; 24.9g protein; 6.5g fibre

Substitute baby spinach leaves for the rocket, if you wish.

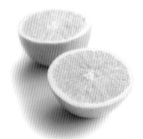

snack 1 medium orange

1 small brown onion (80g), chopped finely
1 clove garlic, crushed
1 tablespoon beef stock
170g lean beef mince
2 small tomatoes (180g), chopped coarsely
¼ teaspoon ground cinnamon
¼ teaspoon ground nutmeg
½ cup (125ml) beef stock, extra
2 tablespoons coarsely chopped fresh flat-leaf parsley
2 tablespoons coarsely chopped fresh basil
1 medium eggplant (300g)
1 small red capsicum (150g), quartered
¼ cup (70g) skim-milk natural yogurt
2 teaspoons finely grated lemon rind
1 tablespoon lemon juice
20g baby rocket leaves

1  Cook onion, garlic and the beef stock in medium frying pan until onion softens. Add beef, tomato and spices; cook, stirring, until beef is browned. Add extra stock; bring to the boil. Reduce heat; simmer, uncovered, about 5 minutes or until liquid is absorbed. Remove from heat; stir in herbs.
2  Meanwhile, slice eggplant lengthways into 6 slices; discard the two outside pieces. Cook eggplant and capsicum on heated grill plate (or grill or barbecue) until browned and tender.
3  Combine yogurt, rind and juice in small jug.
4  Stack beef mixture, eggplant, capsicum and rocket on plates; drizzle with the yogurt mixture.

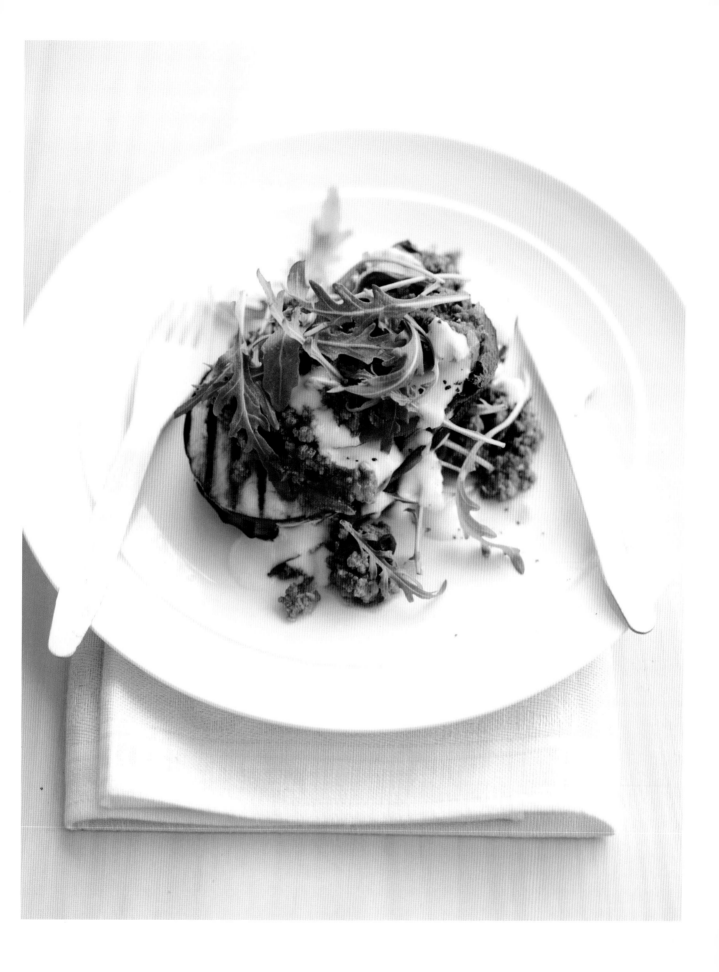

# Day 17 Menu

cranberry and apple muesli | salmon pasta salad | sweet chilli chicken salad

# cranberry and apple muesli

**preparation time** 5 minutes
(plus refrigeration time) **serves** 2
**nutritional count per serving** 3.2g total fat
(0.6g saturated fat); 1133kJ (271 cal);
48.1g carbohydrate; 9.9g protein; 4.1g fibre

**¾ cup (200g) skim-milk natural yogurt**
**¾ cup (65g) rolled oats**
**⅓ cup (80ml) unsweetened apple juice**
**1 small green apple (130g), grated coarsely**
**¼ cup (35g) dried cranberries**

1  Combine yogurt, oats and juice in small bowl;
cover, refrigerate 3 hours or overnight.
2  Just before serving, stir in remaining ingredients.

## Sarah's diary

*Was great to get up this
morning and just pull
breakfast straight from
the fridge – the joys of
preparing it the night before!
Muesli is one of my all-time
favourites, and this one
did not disappoint. Wasn't
actually that hungry at
lunchtime, and just picked
at the salad. Made dinner
for a couple of friends, and
everyone really enjoyed the
salad – I wouldn't mind
taking some to work for
lunch one day.*

## Pamela's diary

*So far, I've lost more weight
than Sarah, the sad truth
is, I had more to lose. Sarah
has been more diligent with
exercise than me during
this diet, maybe she has
developed muscle, whereas
there's very little chance of
that happening to me. I love
to walk, but by nature, I'm
not one to push myself.
However, now that I'm
feeling more energetic due
to the weight loss, I'm up in
the morning, and walking
more and faster than before.*

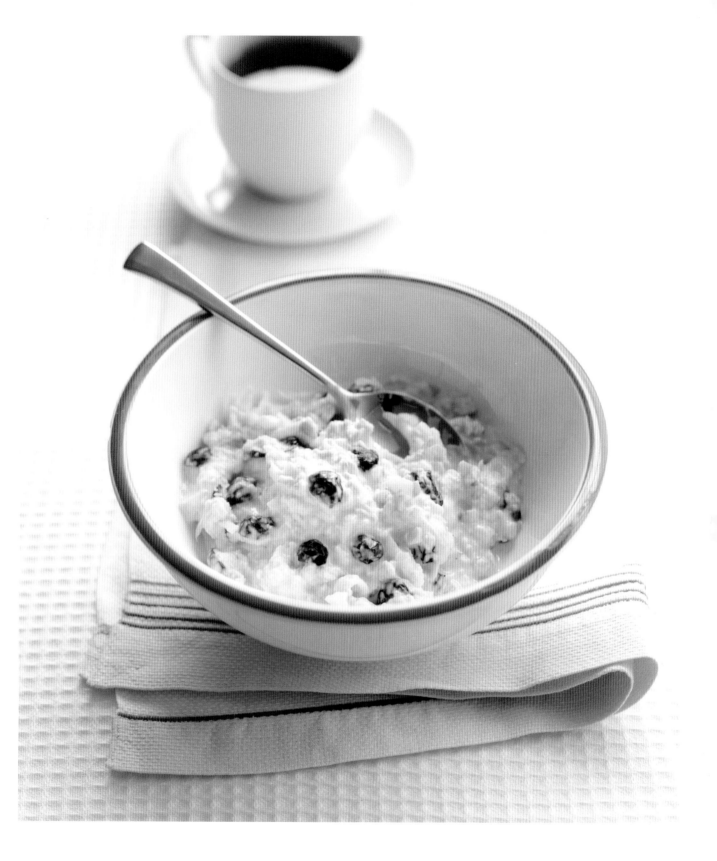

It's not vital that you soak the oats
overnight, but it's preferable.
Cranberries are rich in anti-oxidants,
but if you like, substitute sultanas.

Choose any pasta you like for this delicious salad. You could make it the night before, if you like. Keep it in the fridge.

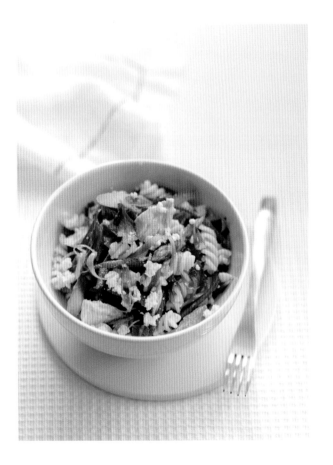

snack 2 cups plain popcorn (see page 52)

preparation time 10 minutes
cooking time 10 minutes  serves 2
nutritional count per serving  8.5g total fat
(2.9g saturated fat); 1860kJ (445 cal);
56.4g carbohydrate; 32.3g protein; 5.1g fibre

LUNCH

# salmon pasta salad

1 cup (150g) spiral pasta
170g asparagus, trimmed, chopped coarsely
2 tablespoons low-fat ricotta cheese
1 teaspoon finely grated lemon rind
¼ cup (60ml) lemon juice
1 clove garlic, crushed
1 small red capsicum (150g), sliced thinly
⅓ cup coarsely chopped fresh flat-leaf parsley
2 green onions, sliced thinly
210g can pink salmon in springwater, drained, flaked

1  Cook pasta in medium saucepan of boiling water, uncovered, until just tender. Add asparagus; cook 1 minute. Drain.
2  Meanwhile, combine cheese, rind, juice and garlic in large bowl; add pasta, asparagus and remaining ingredients to bowl; toss to combine.

# sweet chilli chicken salad

2 cups (500ml) water
200g chicken breast fillet
1¼ cups (100g) bean sprouts
1 small red capsicum (150g), sliced thinly
1 small carrot (70g), cut into matchsticks
1 fresh long red chilli, sliced thinly
⅓ cup firmly packed fresh coriander leaves
3cm piece fresh ginger (15g), cut into matchsticks
¼ cup (60ml) lime juice
1 tablespoon sweet chilli sauce
2 teaspoons fish sauce

**1** Bring water to the boil in medium saucepan; add chicken. Simmer, covered, about 10 minutes or until chicken is cooked. Cool chicken in poaching liquid 10 minutes; drain, shred coarsely.
**2** Combine chicken in medium bowl with sprouts, capsicum, carrot, chilli, coriander and ginger.
**3** Shake juice and sauces together in screw-top jar, drizzle over salad.

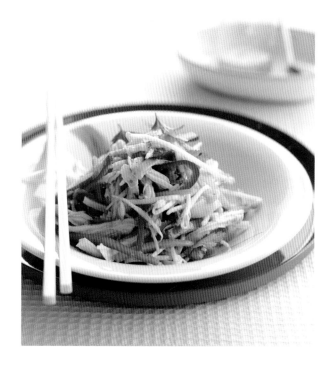

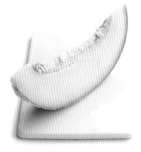

snack 200g rockmelon

**preparation time** 15 minutes
**cooking time** 10 minutes  **serves** 2
**nutritional count per serving**  2.9g total fat
(0.6g saturated fat); 727kJ (174 cal);
8.2g carbohydrate; 26.5g protein; 4.2g fibre

Add a finely chopped fresh red thai chilli if you want to heat up this salad.

# Day 18 Menu  brekky beans | tuna tabbouleh | beef skewers with greek salad

BREAKFAST

# brekky beans

preparation time 10 minutes
cooking time 10 minutes serves 2
nutritional count per serving 2.8g total fat
(0.5g saturated fat); 1241kJ (297 cal);
43.3g carbohydrate; 17.3g protein; 13.4g fibre

1 small brown onion (80g), chopped finely
1 clove garlic, crushed
2 shortcut bacon rashers (30g), chopped finely
400g can diced tomatoes
1 tablespoon tomato paste
1 tablespoon wholegrain mustard
400g can white beans, rinsed, drained
2 tablespoons coarsely chopped fresh flat-leaf parsley
2 slices rye bread (90g), toasted

1  Cook onion, garlic and bacon in heated medium saucepan until onion softens. Add undrained tomatoes, paste and mustard; cook, stirring, until hot. Add beans; cook, stirring, until hot. Stir in parsley.
2  Serve bean mixture with toast.

## Sarah's diary
*I can't believe the diet finishes on Sunday – time has flown. I'm really looking forward to weighing myself at the end. Loved breakfast this morning, I think it's becoming quite obvious what my favourite meal of the day is! Had to eat lunch in a flash because we were so busy, thankfully it was just a light salad, but still delicious.*

## Pamela's diary
*Loved the beans for breakfast, they're so good for the digestive system. Lots of tastings today, both sweet and savoury: it's hard to walk away from food that you really like, but we do keep an eye on each other, which helps. I had to go to a lunch for work today – had to eat three courses, and drank a glass (or was it two?) of Champagne... oh well, someone has to do it.*

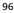

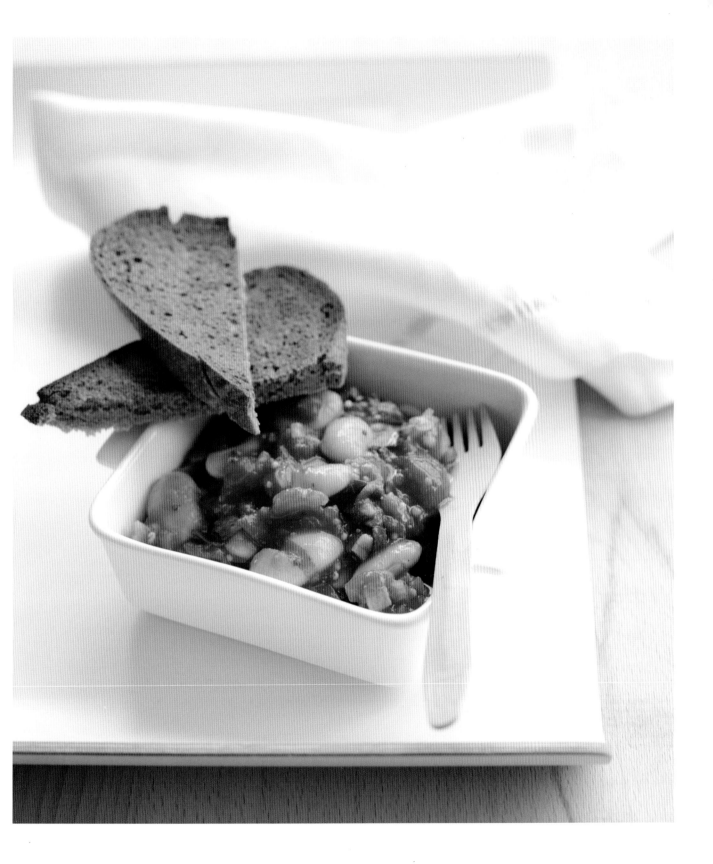

Shortcut bacon is the largest, and
leanest, end of a bacon rasher.
Any canned white bean can be
used; we like cannelini beans.

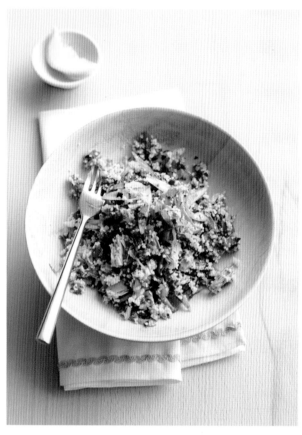

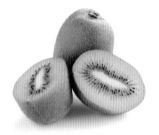

snack 2 kiwifruit

# tuna tabbouleh

**preparation time** 10 minutes  **serves** 2
**nutritional count per serving**  2.4g total fat
(0.8g saturated fat); 920kJ (220 cal);
23.4g carbohydrate; 24.0g protein; 3.2g fibre

¼ cup (50g) couscous
¼ cup (60ml) boiling water
185g can tuna in springwater, drained, flaked
½ cup finely chopped fresh flat-leaf parsley
3 small tomatoes (270g), seeded, chopped finely
3 green onions, sliced thinly
¼ cup (60ml) lemon juice
1 clove garlic, crushed

1  Combine couscous with the water in medium heatproof
bowl, cover; stand 5 minutes or until water is absorbed.
Mix in remaining ingredients.

Make the salad the night
before, or in the morning
and keep it in the fridge.

preparation time 15 minutes
cooking time 10 minutes  serves 2
nutritional count per serving  5.4g total fat
(1.8g saturated fat); 1020kJ (244 cal);
8.7g carbohydrate; 37.8g protein; 4.0g fibre

DINNER

# beef skewers with greek salad

300g rump steak, cut into 2cm cubes
1 tablespoon finely chopped fresh thyme
cooking-oil spray
2 small tomatoes (190g), chopped coarsely
1 small green capsicum (150g), chopped coarsely
¼ cup (30g) seeded black olives
1 lebanese cucumber (130g), chopped coarsely
¼ cup coarsely chopped fresh flat-leaf parsley
1 lemon

1  Combine beef and thyme in medium bowl; thread
beef onto skewers. Spray beef with cooking oil; cook
skewers on heated grill plate (or grill or barbecue).
2  Meanwhile, combine remaining ingredients in
medium bowl.
3  Serve salad with beef skewers and lemon wedges.

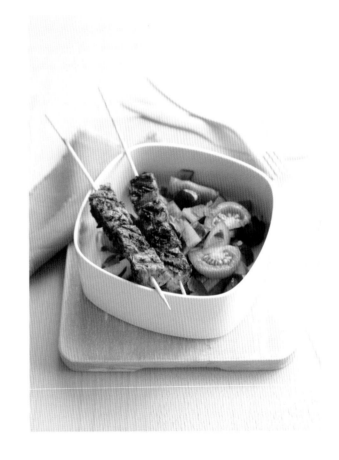

You need to soak four bamboo
skewers in cold water for at least
10 minutes before using to prevent
them scorching during cooking. If
you think of it, overnight soaking
of the bamboo skewers is even
better. You can, of course, use
metal skewers, if you prefer.

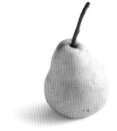

snack 1 small pear

# Day 19 Menu

breakfast fry-up | chicken and bacon club | cajun fish with rice pilaf

# breakfast fry-up

**preparation time** 5 minutes
**cooking time** 10 minutes  **serves** 2
**nutritional count per serving**  1.5g total fat
(0.1g saturated fat); 652kJ (156 cal);
22.5g carbohydrate; 8.9g protein; 7.6g fibre

2 small tomatoes (180g), quartered
1 tablespoon balsamic vinegar
150g mushrooms, sliced thickly
100g baby spinach leaves
2 tablespoons coarsely chopped fresh basil
2 slices rye bread (90g), toasted

**1**  Preheat oven to 220°C/200°C fan-forced.
**2**  Combine tomato and half the vinegar in small shallow baking dish. Roast, uncovered, about 10 minutes.
**3**  Meanwhile, cook mushrooms, spinach and remaining vinegar in large frying pan until mushroom is tender and spinach wilts; stir in basil.
**4**  Serve tomato and mushroom mixture on toast.

It's worth buying the best, most flavoursome tomatoes you can. We use a balsamic vinegar bought from the supermarket, but if you're lucky enough to have a first-grade balsamic vinegar, use it sparingly, as you might only need 1 teaspoon instead of 1 tablespoon.

### Sarah's diary
*Bought a pair of jeans last night, was very exciting – haven't been brave enough to go shopping for jeans for about 3 years. Was super-rushed this morning, so I just had a bowl of the bran & cranberry muesli from Day 4 for breakfast – an easy solution if you're running short of time. The dinner was especially yummy, haven't had pilaf in a long time and it was delicious.*

### Pamela's diary
*Never seen Sarah in jeans before, she looks great, positively leggy. Today's meals were particularly scrumptious; the fry-up seemed decadent, but the fat count has been carefully calculated, you could fool anyone into believing that this is not a diet breakfast. The club sandwich was wonderful, not to mention the fish with a pilaf, oh joy.*

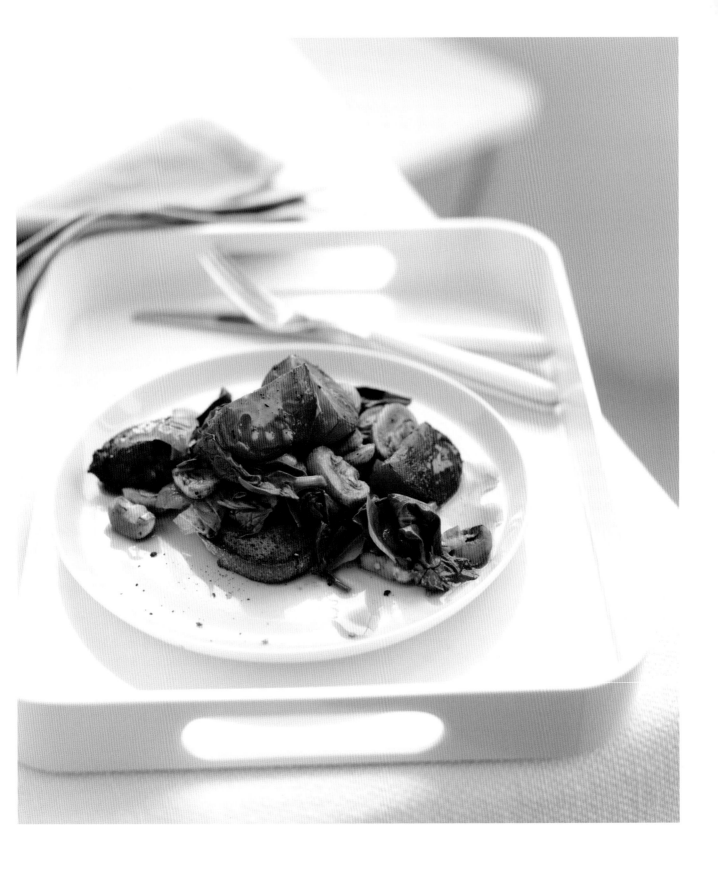

This sandwich is at its best eaten warm, but if you don't have the right facilities to cook the chicken and bacon at lunch time, then cook the chicken and bacon in the morning and assemble the sandwich at work.

snack 125g grapes

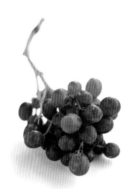

# chicken and bacon club

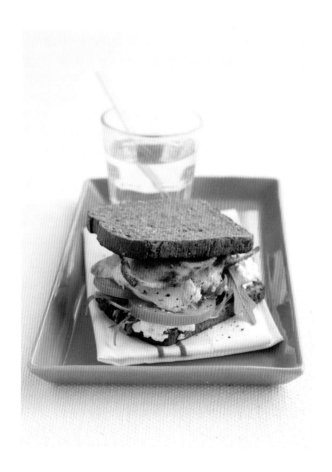

100g chicken breast fillet
cooking-oil spray
2 shortcut bacon rashers (30g)
⅓ cup (65g) low-fat cottage cheese
4 slices rye bread (180g), toasted
20g baby rocket leaves
1 small tomato (90g), sliced thinly

1  Spray chicken with cooking oil; heat medium frying pan, cook chicken. Cover chicken; stand 5 minutes, then slice thinly.
2  Cook bacon in same pan until crisp.
3  Divide half the cheese between two toast slices; top with rocket, tomato, chicken, bacon, remaining cheese and toast.

preparation time 10 minutes
cooking time 8 minutes  serves 2
nutritional count per serving  5.6g total fat
(1.2g saturated fat); 1459kJ (349 cal);
41.5g carbohydrate; 29.1g protein; 6.8g fibre

Choose any white firm-fleshed fish you like; a thick-cut fillet or steak will be best.

# cajun fish with rice pilaf

cooking-oil spray
1 small brown onion (80g), chopped finely
2 trimmed celery stalks (200g), chopped finely
2 cloves garlic, crushed
¼ teaspoon ground cinnamon
2 cloves
¼ teaspoon ground turmeric
¾ cup (150g) white long-grain rice
2 cups (500ml) chicken stock
¼ cup finely chopped fresh flat-leaf parsley
2 x 180g firm white fish fillets
2 teaspoons cajun spice powder

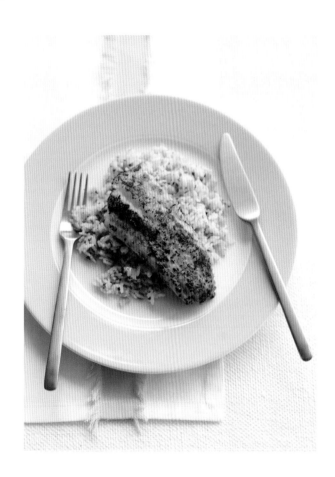

1  Spray base of medium saucepan with cooking oil; cook onion, celery and garlic, stirring, 5 minutes. Add spices; cook, stirring, until fragrant. Add rice; stir to coat in mixture. Add stock; bring to the boil. Reduce heat; simmer, covered tightly, about 20 minutes or until rice is tender and liquid is absorbed. Stir in parsley.
2  Meanwhile, spray medium frying pan with cooking oil. Sprinkle fish with cajun spice; cook in pan.
3  Serve pilaf with fish.

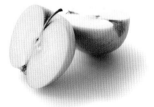

snack 1 small apple

preparation time 10 minutes
cooking time 20 minutes  serves 2
nutritional count per serving  6.6g total fat
(1.9g saturated fat); 2149kJ (514 cal);
64.7g carbohydrate; 46.0g protein; 3.8g fibre

# Day 20 Menu

muesli muffins | tomato, zucchini and oregano slice | teriyaki chicken with noodles

**preparation time** 5 minutes
**cooking time** 25 minutes **makes** 6
**nutritional count per muffin** 9.1g total fat;
2.2g saturated fat; 1756kJ (420 cal);
64.7g carbohydrate; 16.2g protein; 5.7g fibre

### Sarah's diary
*Tomorrow is D-day!
Goodness me…time flies
when you're losing weight!
The muffins were good for
breakfast; I didn't have an
orange so I used lemon rind
instead. Oregano is my
least-favourite herb but,
surprisingly, I enjoyed lunch.
Went out for dinner with
friends; it was quite hard
deciding what to have on
the menu as nothing seemed
particularly healthy…what
can you do. To compensate
for my potentially unhealthy
meal, I didn't have any wine
and didn't even look at the
dessert menu.*

### Pamela's diary
*The reason we decided to
make this diet a 21-day diet
was quite simple, one or two
weeks didn't seem enough,
and if we wanted to go on
it again, the meals would
have seemed repetitive, so,
we decided three weeks was
just right. Sometimes people
diet because they want to lose
a few kilos for an occasion,
or to fit into a certain outfit,
this diet would be ideal for
that reason. But best of all,
because it's not a crash diet,
you won't look drawn or feel
low in energy.*

BREAKFAST

# muesli muffins

cooking-oil spray
½ cup bran and cranberry muesli (see recipe, page 32)
1 teaspoon vegetable oil
½ cup (140g) skim-milk natural yogurt
1 egg
⅔ cup (100g) self-raising flour
2 teaspoons finely grated orange rind
¼ teaspoon mixed spice
1 tablespoon demerara sugar
1 tablespoon low-fat ricotta cheese

1  Preheat oven to 180°C/160°C fan-forced. Spray six ⅓-cup (80ml) muffin pan holes with cooking oil, or line with paper cases.
2  Combine muesli, oil, yogurt, egg, flour, rind and spice in medium bowl, mix with fork.
3  Divide mixture among pan holes; sprinkle with sugar. Bake about 25 minutes.
4  Serve 2 muffins each with cheese.

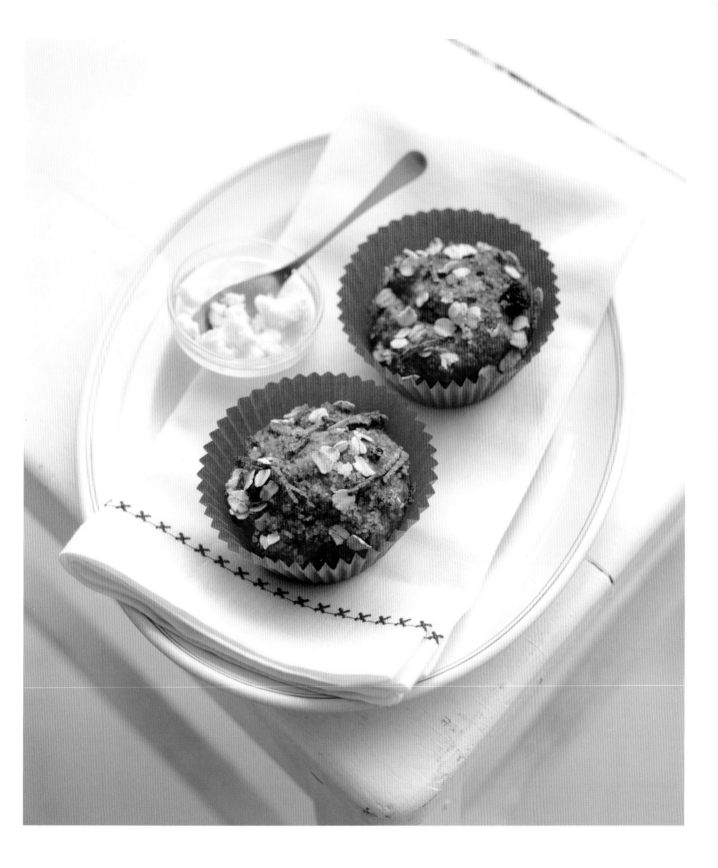

The muffins are suitable to freeze, stored in an airtight container, for up to three months. Use raw sugar instead of demerara if you like. Warm muffins are best; they heat well in a microwave oven – about 20 seconds on HIGH (100%) will be enough.

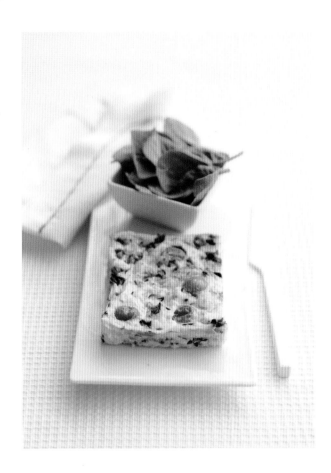

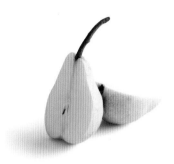

snack 1 small pear

# tomato, zucchini and oregano slice

**preparation time** 10 minutes
**cooking time** 35 minutes **serves** 2
**nutritional count per serving** 3.3g total fat
(1.1g saturated fat); 456kJ (109 cal);
3.1g carbohydrate; 15.7g protein; 2.1g fibre

This slice is great warm
or cold, and can be made
the night before. Keep the
slice in the fridge.

125g cherry tomatoes
1 egg
3 egg whites
⅓ cup (65g) low-fat cottage cheese
1 clove garlic, crushed
1 small zucchini (90g), grated coarsely
2 tablespoons coarsely chopped fresh oregano leaves
30g baby spinach leaves

1  Preheat oven to 200°C/180°C fan-forced. Line an
8cm x 21cm loaf pan with a strip of baking paper.
2  Place tomatoes in pan. Roast 10 minutes.
3  Meanwhile, combine egg, egg whites, cheese and
garlic in medium jug.
4  Remove tomatoes from oven; reduce oven temperature
to 160°C/140°C fan-forced.
5  Sprinkle tomatoes with zucchini and oregano; pour
over egg mixture. Bake about 25 minutes or until set.
6  Serve slice with spinach.

**preparation time** 10 minutes (plus refrigeration time)
**cooking time** 10 minutes  **serves** 2
**nutritional count per serving**  4.3g total fat
(0.8g saturated fat); 1777kJ (425 cal);
59g carbohydrate; 33.7g protein; 5.2g fibre

DINNER

# teriyaki chicken with noodles

160g chicken breast fillet, sliced thinly
⅓ cup (80ml) teriyaki sauce
1 clove garlic, crushed
cooking-oil spray
1 small red onion (100g), cut into wedges
⅓ cup (80ml) chicken stock
200g udon noodles
100g snow peas, halved lengthways
1 cup (80g) bean sprouts
1 fresh small red thai chilli, sliced thinly

**1**  Combine chicken, half the sauce and garlic in medium bowl; cover. Refrigerate 30 minutes.
**2**  Spray wok with cooking oil; cook chicken, in batches, in heated wok until browned.
**3**  Cook onion in wok 1 minute. Return chicken to wok with remaining sauce, stock, noodles and peas; stir-fry until hot.
**4**  Serve stir-fry topped with sprouts and chilli.

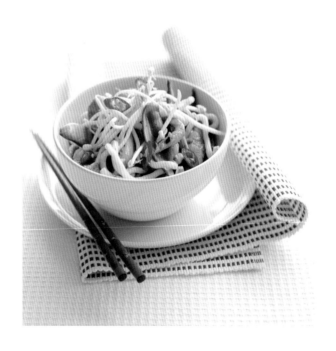

As with all stir-fries, do the preparation before you start to cook. If you don't like chilli, just leave it out.

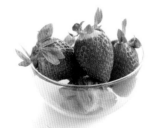

snack 125g strawberries

# Day 21 Menu

egg and bacon pies | chicken and pumpkin tortilla | honey-lemon prawn stir-fry

## egg and bacon pies

preparation time 5 minutes
cooking time 15 minutes serves 2
nutritional count per serving 7.2g total fat
(2.0g saturated fat); 895kJ (214 cal);
21.0g carbohydrate; 21.0g protein; 3.6g fibre

2 shortcut bacon rashers (30g), chopped finely
2 eggs
2 slices rye bread (90g), toasted
1 small tomato (90g), chopped finely

1 Preheat oven to 200°C/180°C fan-forced.
2 Divide bacon between two ⅓-cup (80ml) muffin pan holes. Crack an egg into each hole. Bake, about 15 minutes or until egg is set. Loosen edge of pies from pan.
3 Serves pies on toast, sprinkled with tomato.

### Sarah's diary
*5kg gone! And, it was sooooo easy. I feel fantastic – so fantastic, in fact, that Pamela and I are going to start the diet again tomorrow. Energised, inspired and fresh, I'm ready for another 21 days of good food...and weight loss, too.*

### Pamela's diary
*Not that I'm gloating, but I've lost a whisker under six kilos in the last three weeks and, as I've told you, I've fallen off the diet several times. It is an easy diet to follow; the recipes are easy to make and have been devised to follow nutritional guidelines. It is essentially a low-fat diet, if you follow it, you WILL lose weight, there is no doubt about that. Give it a go, but remember to first check with your health practitioner if you have a medical condition.*

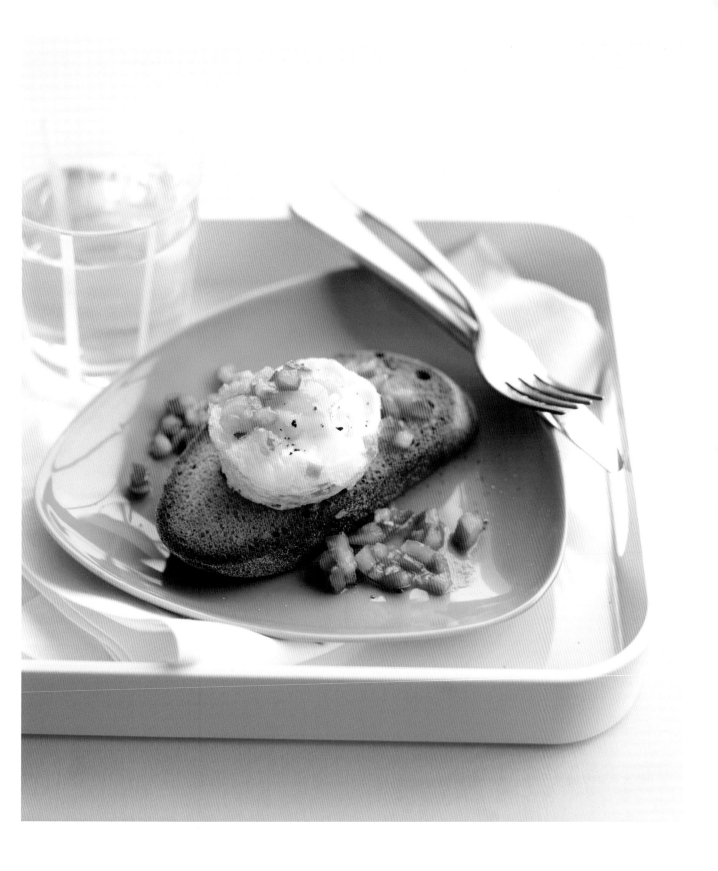

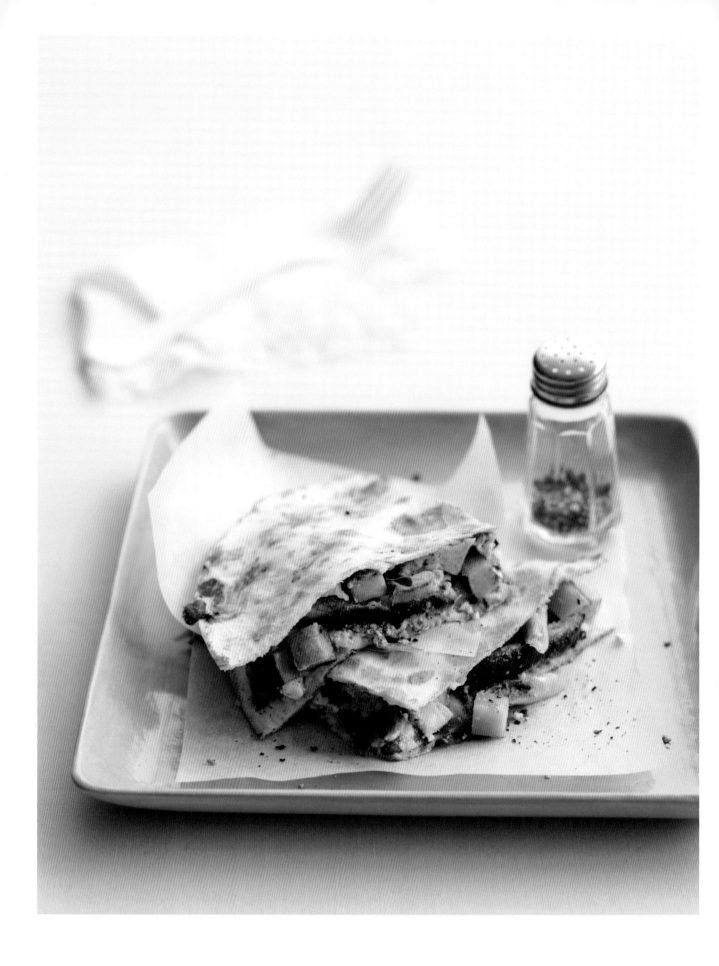

Make the filling the night before, and fill the tortillas in the morning. If you have access to a sandwich press – heat the tortilla in the press.

LUNCH

# chicken and pumpkin tortilla

**preparation time** 10 minutes
**cooking time** 10 minutes  **serves** 2
**nutritional count per serving**  6.4g total fat
(1.5g saturated fat); 1195kJ (286 cal);
26.1g carbohydrate; 29.1g protein; 3.0g fibre

160g chicken breast fillet
1 tablespoon taco seasoning mix
cooking-oil spray
150g butternut pumpkin, cut into 1cm cubes
2 tablespoons coarsely chopped fresh coriander
⅓ cup (65g) low-fat cottage cheese
2 green onions, chopped finely
2 tablespoons lime juice
1 clove garlic, crushed
2 x 15cm flour tortillas

1  Combine chicken and seasoning in small bowl.
2  Spray chicken with cooking oil; cook chicken, on one side, in heated medium frying pan 5 minutes. Turn chicken; add pumpkin. Cook chicken and pumpkin, uncovered, about 5 minutes or until both are cooked.
3  Chop chicken coarsely; combine in medium bowl with pumpkin and coriander.
4  Combine cheese, onion, juice and garlic in small bowl.
5  Spread cheese mixture, then chicken mixture on one tortilla; top with remaining tortilla. Serve cut into wedges.

snack muesli muffin (from day 20)

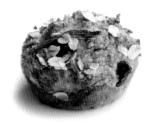

Have everything prepared before you start to cook. If you like, use brown rice instead of white.

DINNER

# honey-lemon prawn stir-fry

**preparation time** 15 minutes
**cooking time** 10 minutes  **serves** 2
**nutritional count per serving** 2.1g total fat
(0.3g saturated fat); 1509kJ (361 cal);
43.8g carbohydrate; 38.6g protein; 4.1g fibre

⅓ cup (65g) white long-grain rice
1 teaspoon sesame seeds
650g uncooked king prawns, shelled,
    deveined, tails intact
1 small brown onion (80g), halved, cut into wedges
300g wombok, sliced thinly
1 small carrot (70g), cut into matchsticks
2 tablespoons lemon juice
1 tablespoon honey
2cm piece fresh ginger (10g), grated
2 green onions, sliced thinly

1  Cook rice in medium saucepan of boiling water, uncovered, until tender; drain.
2  Meanwhile, toast sesame seeds in heated wok; remove from wok.
3  Cook prawns in heated wok; remove.
4  Stir-fry brown onion in heated wok about 3 minutes or until tender. Return prawns to wok with wombok, carrot, juice, honey and ginger; stir-fry until hot.
5  Serve rice with stir-fry, sprinkled with sesame seeds and green onion.

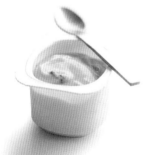

snack 100g skim-milk
fruit-flavoured yogurt

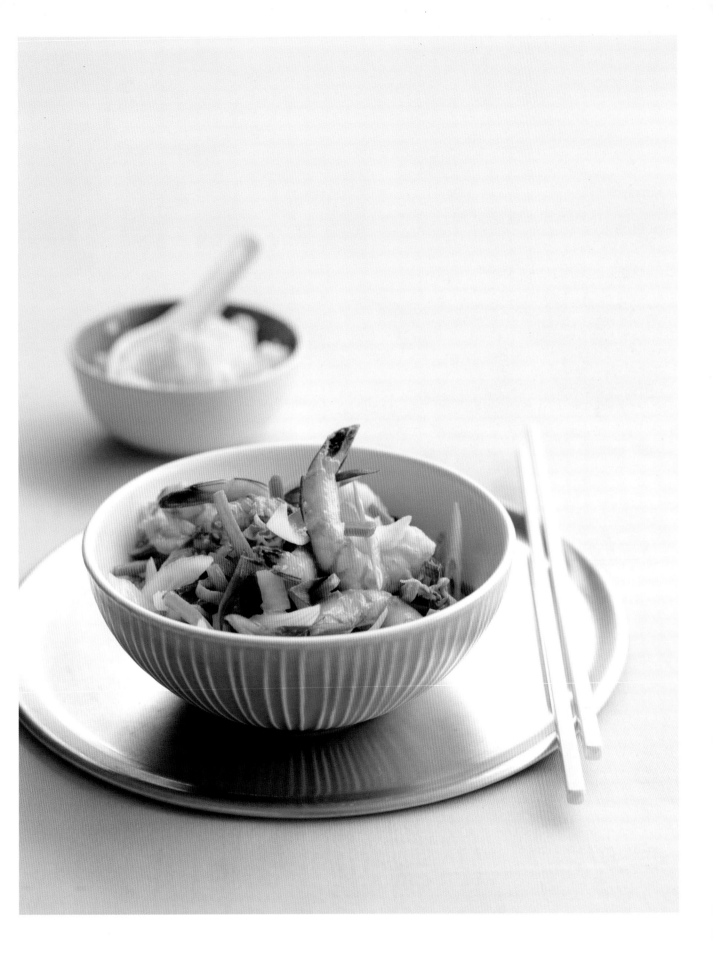

# Shopping List

STAPLES

**PANTRY**
1 can cooking-oil spray
Small bottle
  vegetable oil
Small bottle
  balsamic vinegar
Small jar fat-free
  mayonnaise
1 jar dijon mustard
1 jar wholegrain mustard
500ml beef stock
500ml vegetable stock
1 litre chicken stock
125g can four-bean mix
3 x 125g cans chickpeas
300g can chickpeas
400g can white beans
400g can brown lentils
425g can baby beets
3 x 310g cans corn kernels
5 x 185g cans tuna
  in springwater
210g can salmon
  in springwater
Small can anchovy fillets
2 x 400g cans
  diced tomatoes
Small tub tomato paste
Small can
  light coconut milk
Small bottle
  sweet chilli sauce
Small bottle fish sauce
Small bottle
  teriyaki sauce
Small bottle hoisin sauce
Small bottle oyster sauce
Small bottle
  light soy sauce
Small jar baby capers
Small jar cornichons
Small jar cranberry sauce
Small can green
  peppercorns
Small packet
  sesame seeds

Curry powder
Ground cumin
Dried chilli flakes
Sumac
Tandoori powder
Cajun spice powder
Ground fennel
Ground turmeric
Ground nutmeg
Ground cinnamon
Mixed spice
Whole cloves
Taco seasoning mix
Flour tortillas
Small packet small
  pappadams
Large packet brown rice
Small packet white
  long-grain rice
250g packet couscous
Small packet
  linguine pasta
Small packet spiral pasta
Small packet
  udon noodles (200g)
Small packet rolled oats
Small packet All Bran
Small packet white
  self-raising flour
Small packet wholemeal
  self-raising flour
Small packet brown sugar
Small packet
  demerara sugar
Small jar honey
Packet corn thins
Packet of popping corn
Small packet dried
  cranberries (need 80g)
Small packet dried dates
Small bottle diet
  cranberry juice

**FREEZER**
Small packet frozen
  baby peas

SHOPPING LIST WEEK 1

**FRIDGE**
5 x 100g tubs skim-milk
  fruit-flavoured yogurt
2 x 140g tubs skim-milk
  natural yogurt
1 x 200g carton low-fat
  ricotta cheese
1 x 200g tub low-fat
  cottage cheese
600ml carton buttermilk
600ml carton skim milk
12 eggs

**FRUIT & VEG**
600g rockmelon
200g honeydew melon
200g watermelon
1 medium mango
1 punnet blueberries
4 apricots, plums or
  kiwifruit
4 small apples
2 small bananas
250g grapes
5 lemons
2 limes
4 oranges
2 small pears
250g strawberries
5 small tomatoes
125g cherry tomatoes
125g yellow tear drop
  tomatoes
3 small red capsicums
1 fresh small
  red thai chilli
1 fresh long red chilli
1 bunch basil
1 bunch mint
2 bunches coriander
2 bunches flat-leaf parsley
160g baby spinach leaves
170g baby rocket
1 bunch green onions
1 bunch red radishes
  (300g)
150g snow peas

4 passionfruit
1 baby buk choy
170g asparagus
100g green beans
2 lebanese cucumbers
¼ cabbage (80g)
4 small zucchinis (360g)
4 small carrots
2 flat mushrooms (160g)
200g butternut pumpkin
650g kumara
6 baby new potatoes (240g)
2 small brown onions
4 small red onions
1 bulb garlic
  (need 10 cloves)

**MEAT & SEAFOOD**
200g chicken breast fillet
280g chicken tenderloins
4 french-trimmed lamb
  cutlets (200g)
180g beef rump steak
2 pork cutlets (280g)
180g lean beef mince
320g white fish fillets
400g marinara mix
75g shaved ham
4 slices (120g) rare
  roast beef

**MISCELLANEOUS**
1 packet multi-grain
  english muffins
1 small loaf rye bread
1 packet rye mountain
  bread wraps

This comprehensive list covers every ingredient in the 21-day diet; most of the staples will be in your pantry already.

## SHOPPING LIST WEEK 2

**FRIDGE**
8 x 100g tubs skim-milk
  fruit-flavoured yogurt
1 x 140g tub skim-milk
  natural yogurt
1 x 200g tub low-fat
  cottage cheese
2 x 200g cartons low-fat
  ricotta cheese
30g reduced-fat
  feta cheese
600ml carton skim milk
600ml carton buttermilk
12 eggs

**FRUIT & VEG**
800g watermelon
500g strawberries
75g blueberries
135g raspberries
1 ruby-red grapefruit
6 small bananas
2 small apples
3 small pears
4 kiwifruit
2 medium oranges
4 passionfruit
250g grapes
3 lemons
4 limes
6 small tomatoes
3 small red capsicums
2 fresh small
  red thai chillies
2 fresh long red chillies
1 bunch basil
2 bunches mint
1 bunch dill
1 bunch chives
2 bunches coriander
2 bunches flat-leaf parsley
30g baby rocket
60g baby spinach leaves
30g snow pea sprouts
2 bunches green onions
  (need 16 onions)
2 lebanese cucumbers

½ bunch celery
  (need 6 stalks)
150g green beans
1 iceberg lettuce
2 cobs corn
115g baby corn
80g bean sprouts
350g watercress
170g asparagus
175g broccolini
3 small carrots
4 flat mushrooms (320g)
3 small red onions
400g kipfler potatoes
1 medium kumara (400g)
150g butternut pumpkin
Ginger (about 35g knob)
1 bulb garlic
  (need 8 cloves)

**MEAT & SEAFOOD**
600g chicken breast fillet
200g lamb backstrap
200g beef rump steak
2 beef eye-fillet
  steaks (250g)
220g lean beef mince
250g pork fillet
30g sliced prosciutto
80g shaved turkey
300g firm white fish fillets
250g small cooked prawns
150g shaved ham

**MISCELLANEOUS**
1 small loaf rye bread
1 packet rye mountain
  bread wraps
1 packet large wholemeal
  pitta bread

## SHOPPING LIST WEEK 3

**FRIDGE**
1 x 200g tub skim-milk
  passionfruit-flavoured
  yogurt
4 x 100g tubs skim-milk
  fruit-flavoured yogurt
4 x 140g tubs skim-milk
  natural yogurt
1 x 200g carton low-fat
  ricotta cheese
1 x 250g tub low-fat
  cottage cheese
600ml carton skim milk
8 eggs
Small carton unsweetened
  apple juice

**FRUIT & VEG**
310g strawberries
2 medium bananas (400g)
5 small apples
4 small pears
400g rockmelon
250g grapes
4 kiwifruit
1 medium
  pink grapefruit (425g)
5 medium oranges
6 lemons
4 limes
250g grape tomatoes
125g cherry tomatoes
11 small tomatoes
3 small red capsicums
1 small green capsicum
3 lebanese cucumbers
1 medium eggplant (300g)
1 fresh small
  red thai chilli
1 fresh long red chilli
1 bunch fresh thyme
1 bunch oregano
1 bunch basil
1 bunch dill
4 bunches flat-leaf parsley
1 bunch coriander
1 bunch green onions

1 bunch chives
150g baby spinach leaves
40g baby rocket
2 baby cos lettuce
170g asparagus
1 small zucchini
½ bunch celery
  (need 4 stalks)
300g wombok
180g bean sprouts
100g snow peas
4 small brown onions
2 small red onions
150g mushrooms
150g butternut pumpkin
2 small carrots
3 medium potatoes (400g)
Ginger (need 30g knob)
1 bulb garlic
  (need 9 cloves)

**MEAT & SEAFOOD**
880g chicken breast fillet
300g beef rump steak
170g lean beef mince
6 shortcut bacon rashers
30g sliced prosciutto
360g firm white fish fillets
650g uncooked
  king prawns

**MISCELLANEOUS**
1 x 800g loaf rye bread
30g black olives

# Glossary

**ALL-BRAN** A cereal made from wheat bran.

**BABY BEETS** Whole canned baby beetroot; also known as red beets.

**BALSAMIC VINEGAR** Deep rich brown vinegar made from Trebbiano grapes; has a sweet/sour flavour.

**BABY BUK CHOY** Sometimes called shanghai buk choy or white cabbage (pak kat farang); has a mildly acrid, distinctively appealing taste.

**BACON, SHORTCUT** Is a "half rasher"; the streaky (belly), narrow portion of the rasher has been removed leaving the choice cut eye meat (rounded end).

**BASIL** An aromatic herb; there are many types, but the most commonly used is sweet, or common, basil.

**BEANS**
**four bean mix** Made up of kidney beans, butter beans, chickpeas and great northern beans.
**sprouts** Also known as bean shoots; tender new growths of assorted beans and seeds germinated for consumption as sprouts. The most readily available are mung bean, soybean, alfalfa and snow pea sprouts. Sprout mixtures or tendrils are also available.
**white** A generic term we use for canned or dried cannellini, haricot, navy or great northern beans.

**BREAD**
**english muffin** A round teacake made from yeast, flour, milk, semolina and salt; often confused with crumpets. Pre-baked and sold packaged in supermarkets, muffins should be split open and toasted before eating.
**pitta** Also known as lebanese bread; wheat-flour pocket bread sold in large, flat pieces that separate into two thin rounds. Also available in small thick pieces called pocket pitta.
**rye** Made with or partly with rye flour. It can be light or dark in colour.
**rye mountain wraps** Flat, thin, soft-textured, yeast-free bread made from wholemeal rye and wheaten flour; available from supermarkets.

**tortilla** Thin, round unleavened bread originating in Mexico. Two kinds are available, one made from wheat flour and the other from corn.

**BROCCOLINI** A cross between broccoli and chinese kale; long asparagus-like stems with a long loose floret, both completely edible. Resembles broccoli in look, but milder and sweeter in taste.

**BUTTERMILK** Originally the term given to the slightly sour liquid left after butter was churned from cream, today it is commercially made similarly to yogurt. Sold alongside all fresh milk products in supermarkets; despite the implication of its name, it is low in fat.

**CAPERS** The grey-green buds of a warm climate (usually Mediterranean) shrub, sold either dried and salted or pickled in a vinegar brine. Baby capers are also available. Capers should be rinsed well before using.

**CAPSICUM** Also known as bell pepper or, simply, pepper; can be green, yellow, red, orange or purplish-black. Discard seeds and membranes before use.

**CHICKPEAS** Also called garbanzos, hummus or channa; an irregularly round, sandy-coloured legume.

**CORIANDER** Also known as cilantro, pak chee or chinese parsley; a bright-green-leafed herb with a pungent flavour. Both stems and roots are also used in Thai cooking; wash well before chopping. Also available as seeds or ground; these must never be used to replace fresh coriander or vice versa, as the tastes are completely different.

**CORNICHONS** French for gherkin, a very small variety of cucumber.

**COUSCOUS** A fine, grain-like cereal product made from semolina; it is rehydrated by steaming or with the addition of a warm liquid and swells to three or four times its original size.

**CHEESE**
**cottage** Fresh, white, unripened curd cheese with a lumpy consistency and a mild, sweet flavour.

**fetta** A crumbly goat- or sheep-milk cheese having a sharp, salty taste.
**ricotta** Sweet, moist, white cow-milk cheese with a slightly grainy texture.

**CORN THINS** A thin crispbread made from corn; 97% fat free.

**DRIED SWEETENED CRANBERRIES** Also known as craisins. Can usually be substituted for or with other dried fruit in most recipes.

**FISH FILLETS, FIRM WHITE** Any firm boneless fish fillet, such as blue-eye, ling and snapper, are suitable to use.

**KIPFLER POTATOES** Small, finger-shaped potato with a nutty flavour.

**LEBANESE CUCUMBER** Short, slender and thin-skinned. Has tender, edible skin, tiny, yielding seeds and a sweet, fresh and flavoursome taste.

**LENTILS** Dried pulses often identified by and named after their colour (red, brown, yellow); also known as dhal.

**LINGUINE** Known as flat spaghetti or little tongues because of its long, narrow shape.

**MARINARA MIX** A mix of uncooked, chopped seafood; available from fish markets and fishmongers.

**MINCE** Also known as ground meat.

**MUSHROOMS** If a recipe calls for an unspecified type of mushroom, use button, a small, cultivated white mushroom with a mild flavour.
**flat** Large and flat with a rich earthy flavour. Are sometimes misnamed field mushrooms, which are wild mushrooms.

**MUSTARD**
**dijon** Also known as french. Pale brown, creamy, distinctively flavoured, fairly mild French mustard.
**wholegrain** Also known as seeded. A French-style coarse-grain mustard made from crushed mustard seeds and dijon-style french mustard.

**OIL**
**cooking-oil spray** Use a cholesterol-free cooking spray made from canola oil.
**vegetable** Sourced from plants.

**OREGANO, FRESH** Also known as wild marjoram; has a woody stalk with clumps of tiny, dark green leaves that have a pungent, peppery aroma. Related to the mint family.

**PARSLEY, FLAT-LEAF** Also known as continental or italian parsley.

**PAPPADUMS** Dried cracker-like wafers made from a combination of lentil and rice flours, oil and spices.

**PRAWNS** Also known as shrimp.

**PROSCIUTTO** A kind of unsmoked Italian ham; salted, air-cured and aged, it is usually eaten uncooked.

**ROCKET** Also known as arugula, rugula and rucola; a peppery-tasting green leaf that can be used similarly to baby spinach leaves. Baby rocket leaves are both smaller and less peppery.

**ROLLED OATS** Flattened oat grain rolled into flakes and traditionally used for porridge. Instant oats are also available, but use traditional oats for baking.

**SAUCES**
**cranberry** Made of cranberries cooked in sugar syrup.
**fish** Also called naam pla or nuoc naam. Made from pulverised salted fermented fish (most often anchovies); has a pungent smell and strong taste, so use according to your taste.
**hoisin** A thick, sweet and spicy Chinese sauce made from salted fermented soybeans, onions and garlic. From Asian food shops and supermarkets.
**oyster** A thick, richly flavoured brown sauce made from oysters and their brine, and cooked with salt and soy sauce, and thickened with starches.
**soy, japanese** An all-purpose low-salt soy sauce made with more wheat than its Chinese counterparts; fermented in barrels and aged.
**soy, light** Fairly thin, pale and salty tasting; used in dishes in which the natural colour of the ingredients is to be maintained.
**sweet chilli** Mild tasting sauce made from red chillies, sugar, garlic and white wine vinegar.

**teriyaki** A Japanese sauce made from mirin, sugar, soy sauce, ginger and other spices.

**SPICES**
**cajun** A blend of herbs and spices including basil, paprika, tarragon, onion, fennel, thyme and cayenne.
**cinnamon** Dried inner bark of the shoots of the cinnamon tree; available in stick (quill) or ground form.
**cloves** Dried flower buds of a tropical tree; can be used whole or in ground form. Has a distinctively pungent and "spicy" scent and flavour.
**cumin** Also known as zeera or comino; has a spicy, nutty flavour. Available in seed form or dried and ground.
**curry powder** A blend of ground spices including dried chilli, cinnamon, mace, coriander, cumin, fennel, fenugreek, cardamom and turmeric. Choose mild or hot to suit your taste and the recipe.
**fennel, ground** Dried seeds having a licorice flavour, ground to a fine powder.
**green peppercorns** The soft, under-ripe berry that's usually preserved in brine. Has a fresh flavour that's less pungent than the berry in its other forms.
**mixed spice** A blend of ground spices usually consisting of cinnamon, allspice and nutmeg.
**nutmeg** The dried nut of an evergreen tree; it is available ground, or you can grate your own with a fine grater.
**sumac** A purple-red, astringent spice ground from berries growing on wild shrubs found in the Mediterranean; adds a tart, lemony flavour.
**taco seasoning mix** A packaged seasoning meant to duplicate the Mexican sauce made from oregano, cumin, chillies and other spices.
**tandoori spice mix** A blend of spices that imparts the well-known tandoori flavour from India. Includes paprika, cumin, coriander, turmeric, ginger, cinnamon, fenugreek, pepper, chilli, cardamom, caraway and spearmint.
**turmeric** Known for the golden colour it imparts to the dishes of which it's a part. Dried turmeric has a rich, woody aroma and a slightly bitter, musky taste.

**SPINACH** Also known as english spinach and, incorrectly, silver beet.

**STOCK** Available in cans, bottles or tetra packs and as cubes, powder or concentrated liquid. As a guide, 1 teaspoon of stock powder or 1 small crumbled stock cube mixed with 1 cup (250ml) water will give a fairly strong stock. Be aware of the salt and fat content of these stocks.

**SUGAR**
**brown** Soft, finely granulated sugar retaining molasses for its characteristic colour and flavour.
**demerara** Golden-coloured, small-grained crystal sugar.

**THYME, FRESH** A basic herb of French cuisine; a member of the mint family, it has tiny grey-green leaves that give off a pungent minty, light-lemon aroma.

**TOMATOES**
**cherry** A very small, round tomato.
**egg** Also called plum or roma; are smallish, oval-shaped tomatoes.
**paste** Triple-concentrated tomato puree.
**yellow teardrop** A very small, yellow pear-shaped tomato.

**UDON NOODLES** Available fresh and dried, these broad, white Japanese wheat noodles are similar to the ones in homemade chicken noodle soup.

**WATERCRESS** Also known as winter rocket; a slightly peppery, dark-green leaf vegetable. Highly perishable, so use as soon as possible after purchase.

**WOMBOK** Also known as chinese cabbage, peking or napa cabbage; elongated in shape with pale green, crinkly leaves.

**YOGURT**
**skim-milk fruit-flavoured yogurt** We used fruit-flavoured yogurt made with skim milk and sweetened artificially.
**skim-milk natural yogurt** We used natural yogurt with a fat content of less than 0.2 per cent.

**ZUCCHINI** also known as courgette; small green, yellow or white vegetable belonging to the squash family.

# Conversion chart

## MEASURES

One Australian metric measuring cup holds approximately 250ml; one Australian metric tablespoon holds 20ml; one Australian metric teaspoon holds 5ml.

The difference between one country's measuring cups and another's is within a two- or three-teaspoon variance, and will not affect your cooking results. North America, New Zealand and the United Kingdom use a 15ml tablespoon.

All cup and spoon measurements are level. The most accurate way of measuring dry ingredients is to weigh them. When measuring liquids, use a clear glass or plastic jug with the metric markings.

We use large eggs with an average weight of 60g.

## DRY MEASURES

| METRIC | IMPERIAL |
|---|---|
| 15g | ½oz |
| 30g | 1oz |
| 60g | 2oz |
| 90g | 3oz |
| 125g | 4oz (¼lb) |
| 155g | 5oz |
| 185g | 6oz |
| 220g | 7oz |
| 250g | 8oz (½lb) |
| 280g | 9oz |
| 315g | 10oz |
| 345g | 11oz |
| 375g | 12oz (¾lb) |
| 410g | 13oz |
| 440g | 14oz |
| 470g | 15oz |
| 500g | 16oz (1lb) |
| 750g | 24oz (1½lb) |
| 1kg | 32oz (2lb) |

## LIQUID MEASURES

| METRIC | IMPERIAL |
|---|---|
| 30ml | 1 fluid oz |
| 60ml | 2 fluid oz |
| 100ml | 3 fluid oz |
| 125ml | 4 fluid oz |
| 150ml | 5 fluid oz (¼ pint/1 gill) |
| 190ml | 6 fluid oz |
| 250ml | 8 fluid oz |
| 300ml | 10 fluid oz (½ pint) |
| 500ml | 16 fluid oz |
| 600ml | 20 fluid oz (1 pint) |
| 1000ml (1 litre) | 1¾ pints |

## LENGTH MEASURES

| METRIC | IMPERIAL |
|---|---|
| 3mm | ⅛ in |
| 6mm | ¼in |
| 1cm | ½in |
| 2cm | ¾in |
| 2.5cm | 1in |
| 5cm | 2in |
| 6cm | 2½in |
| 8cm | 3in |
| 10cm | 4in |
| 13cm | 5in |
| 15cm | 6in |
| 18cm | 7in |
| 20cm | 8in |
| 23cm | 9in |
| 25cm | 10in |
| 28cm | 11in |
| 30cm | 12in (1ft) |

## OVEN TEMPERATURES

These oven temperatures are only a guide for conventional ovens. For fan-forced ovens, check the manufacturer's manual.

| | °C (CELSIUS) | °F (FAHRENHEIT) | GAS MARK |
|---|---|---|---|
| Very slow | 120 | 250 | ½ |
| Slow | 150 | 275-300 | 1-2 |
| Moderately slow | 160 | 325 | 3 |
| Moderate | 180 | 350-375 | 4-5 |
| Moderately hot | 200 | 400 | 6 |
| Hot | 220 | 425-450 | 7-8 |
| Very hot | 240 | 475 | 9 |

# Index

# If you like this cookbook, you'll love these...

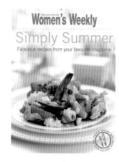
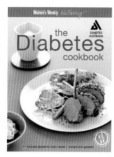
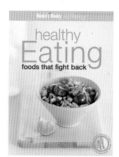

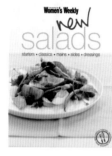
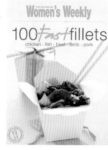
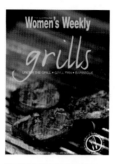

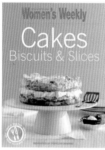
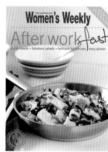
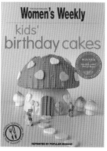

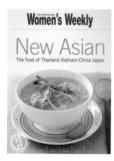
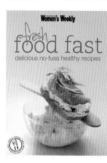
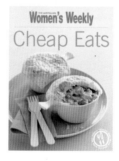

These are just a small selection of titles available in
*The Australian Women's Weekly* range on sale at selected
newsagents, supermarkets or online at www.acpbooks.com.au

# also available in bookstores...

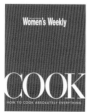
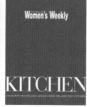
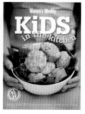

**TEST KITCHEN**
**Food director** Pamela Clark
**Recipe consultant** Sarah Schwikkard
**Test Kitchen manager** Kellie-Marie Thomas
**Home economist** Amanda Lennon
**Nutritional information** Belinda Farlow

**ACP BOOKS**
**General manager** Christine Whiston
**Editorial director** Susan Tomnay
**Creative director & designer** Hieu Chi Nguyen
**Senior editor** Wendy Bryant
**Director of sales** Brian Cearnes
**Marketing manager** Bridget Cody
**Business analyst** Ashley Davies
**Operations manager** David Scotto
**International rights enquires** Laura Bamford
lbamford@acpuk.com

ACP Books are published by ACP Magazines
a division of PBL Media Pty Limited
**Group publisher, Women's lifestyle**
Pat Ingram
**Director of sales, Women's lifestyle**
Lynette Phillips
**Commercial manager, Women's lifestyle**
Seymour Cohen
**Marketing director, Women's lifestyle**
Matthew Dominello
**Public relations manager, Women's lifestyle**
Hannah Deveraux
**Creative director, Events, Women's lifestyle**
Luke Bonnano
**Research Director, Women's lifestyle**
Justin Stone
**ACP Magazines, Chief Executive officer**
Scott Lorson
**PBL Media, Chief Executive officer**
Ian Law

**Produced by** ACP Books, Sydney.
**Published by** ACP Books, a division of
ACP Magazines Ltd, 54 Park St, Sydney;
GPO Box 4088, Sydney, NSW 2001.
phone (02) 9282 8618  fax (02) 9267 9438.
acpbooks@acpmagazines.com.au
www.acpbooks.com.au
**Printed by** Dai Nippon in Korea.

**Australia** Distributed by Network Services,
phone +61 2 9282 8777 fax +61 2 9264 3278
networkweb@networkservicescompany.com.au
**United Kingdom** Distributed by Australian
Consolidated Press (UK),
phone (01604) 642 200 fax (01604) 642 300
books@acpuk.com
**New Zealand** Distributed by Netlink
Distribution Company,
phone (9) 366 9966 ask@ndc.co.nz
**South Africa** Distributed by PSD Promotions,
phone (27 11) 392 6065/6/7
fax (27 11) 392 6079/80
orders@psdprom.co.za

21 day wonder diet: the Australian
women's weekly.
Includes index.
ISBN  978 1 86396 741 9 (pbk).
1. Reducing diets – Recipes. I. Clark, Pamela.
II Title: Australian Women's Weekly
641.5635
© ACP Magazines Ltd 2008
ABN 18 053 273 546
This publication is copyright. No part of it may be
reproduced or transmitted in any form without the
written permission of the publishers.

The publishers would like to thank the following
for props used in photography: Accoutrement,
Alfresco Emporium, Village Living, Mud Australia,
Wheel & Barrow Warringah Mall.
**To order books,**
**phone 136 116 (within Australia).**
**Send recipe enquiries to:**
recipeenquiries@acpmagazines.com.au

# BRIGHTC

Text by
ANGELA FIDDES

Photographs by
ERNEST FRANKL

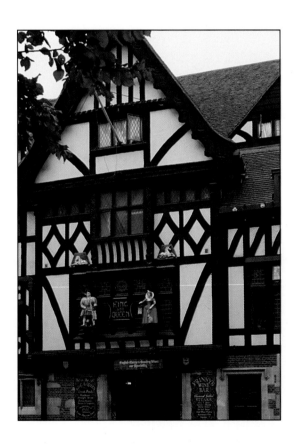

PEVENSEY
*Heritage Guides*

# Brighton

For more than 200 years people have been enjoying the seaside sparkle of Brighton. It has a long beach, with sand at low tide, a big and lively pier, and every facility for sport and amusement. But as its nickname 'London-by-the-Sea' implies, Brighton is a cultural centre as well. At the end of the 18th century the Prince Regent, later George IV, built his exotic Royal Pavilion here and made Brighton a town where all the arts could flourish – music, theatre, painting and architecture. The annual Brighton Festival carries on Prinny's artistic tradition today, while as a contrast yachtsmen will find in Brighton's huge Marina the nearest thing to St Tropez the South Coast has to offer. Each summer, more than 100 yachts gather offshore to race to Fecamp in Normandy, retracing the journey made by the fugitive Charles II after the Battle of Worcester.

## PLACES TO SEE

### A Regency Square

As its name suggests, Regency Square is a typical layout from the heyday of the Prince Regent's building programme. It is spaciously planned round three sides of a green open space.

### B Old Ship Hotel

The hotel, in simple classical style, stands on a site where there has been an inn or hotel since Elizabethan times.

### C The Lanes

The medieval fishing village of Brighthelmstone was bounded by the seafront, West Street, North Street and East Street. About a quarter of this attractively haphazard warren of narrow old streets now forms the area nicknamed the Lanes, where visitors can browse among antique shops, jewellers and boutiques. Scattered among the shops are some of the town's oldest Nonconformist chapels, going back to the 17th century. Look out also for the former House of Correction, built in William IV's time.

### D St Peter's Church

### E St Nicholas's Church

West Pier

### F Palace Pier

The white-painted pier, a quarter of a mile long, was built in the 1890s, some 70 years after the original Chain Pier.

### G Sea Life Centre

*All year, daily. Adm charge.*
*Tel (0273) 604233*

### H Art Gallery and Museum

*All year, daily except Wed. Free entry.*
*Tel (0273) 603005.*
*All year, daily. Adm charge.*
*Tel (0273) 604233*

### I Pelham Square

### J Volk's Electric Railway

Near the entrance to the Palace Pier is the tiny terminus building, hardly larger than a hut, of Britain's first electric-powered railway. It was constructed in 1883 by the Brighton electrical pioneer Magnus Volk, and runs along the seafront for about a mile.
*Apr-Sept, daily. Fares.*
*Tel (0273) 681061.*

Booth Museum 1

A 259
Hove 1
Worthing 12

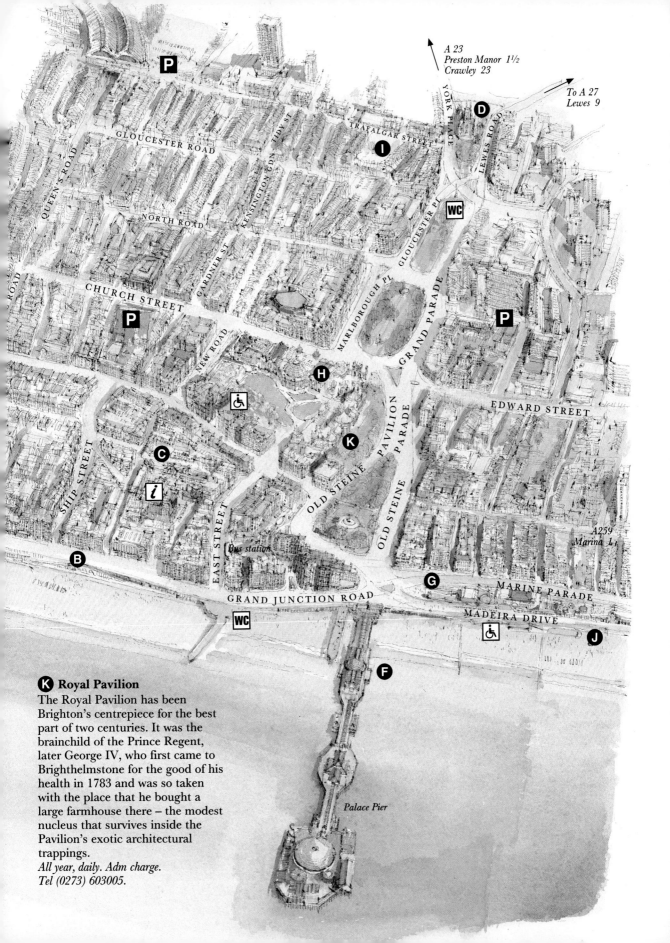

**K Royal Pavilion**

The Royal Pavilion has been Brighton's centrepiece for the best part of two centuries. It was the brainchild of the Prince Regent, later George IV, who first came to Brighthelmstone for the good of his health in 1783 and was so taken with the place that he bought a large farmhouse there – the modest nucleus that survives inside the Pavilion's exotic architectural trappings.

*All year, daily. Adm charge.*
*Tel (0273) 603005.*

A Pevensey Heritage Guide

First published 1983
Reprinted 1989
Revised Edition 1993

Photographs: Ernest Frankl, except front cover, 4, 18: The Royal Pavilion Art Gallery and Museums,
Brighton; 40: Grand Hotel, Brighton; 53: The Brighton Centre

Colour map copyright © The Reader's Digest Association Ltd
Other maps by Carmen Frankl

A catalogue record for this book is available from the British Library.

ISBN 0 907115 60 8

Design by Book Production Consultants, Cambridge
Printed in Hong Kong by Wing King Tong Co. Ltd
for David & Charles plc
Brunel House  Newton Abbot  Devon

The Pevensey Press is an imprint of David & Charles plc

*Front cover*
The Royal Pavilion, east front

*Back cover*
Brighton beach; Regency Square; Meeting House Lane

*Title page inset*
The King and Queen Inn, Marlborough Place

# Contents

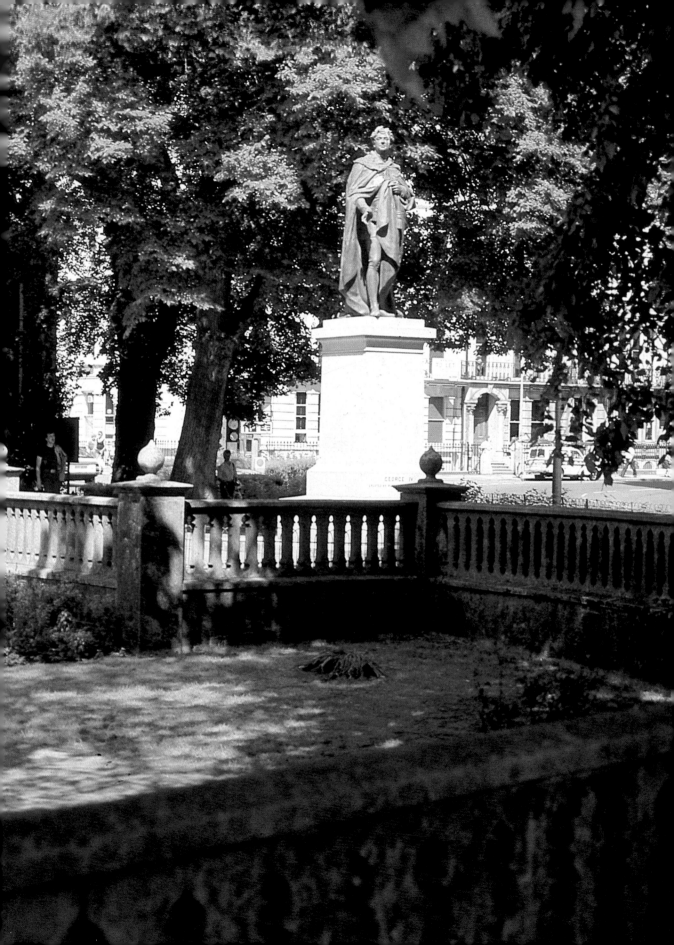

# From Prehistory to the Present

There have been settlements in and around Brighton since Neolithic times, early man preferring to live on high ground such as Whitehawk Hill or Hollingbury Hill, rather than the narrow strip of coastal plain where the modern town centre lies. According to local annals, in Saxon times Brighton was held by Ulnoth, grandfather of King Harold; but it is with the Domesday Book (1086) that our detailed knowledge of 'Bristelmestune', as it calls the settlement, begins. The town's name has changed more than once – for long it was known as Brighthelmeston, the modern form being officially established only in the early 19th century.

In 1086 'Bristelmestune' was a fishing community of about 90 people at the mouth of the Wellesbourne, paying the Crown an annual rent of 4000 herrings. The medieval town consisted of an upper part, inhabited by farmers and artisans, and a lower part, on the beach below the cliff, where fishing families lived. The church of St Nicholas of Myra, the patron saint of fishermen, was built in the 14th century to replace an earlier structure. Its site, on a high hill then outside the town, was chosen either as providing a landmark for sailors, or because of some former pagan association of the hill. Medieval Brighton seems not to have been particularly prosperous. Although in 1313 Edward II granted the right to hold a weekly market (on Thursdays) and a 3-day St Bartholomew fair, the townspeople claimed exemption from taxation in 1349 on the grounds that 'here are no merchants, but tenants of land, who live by their own hand and great labours only'.

The earliest map of Brighton supposedly depicts an attack by the French in 1545 (though it is not certain that this actually took place); it shows that East St, Middle St, West St and North St are survivals of the original rectangular Tudor layout. The area between Middle St and East St was known as the Hempshares: here hemp was grown for the fishermen's nets. Like other south-coast towns Brighton was vulnerable to attack and, in wars against France, to invasion. During the 16th century defences were organised, but not until the town had been almost wholly destroyed. In June 1514 French forces under the notorious admiral Prégent de Bidoux (known in England as 'Prior John') landed and fired the town, seizing what they could before being driven off by a local force hastily summoned by the lighting of beacons on the Downs. All the medieval buildings perished except St Nicholas' church, though the present-day Lanes give some idea of the layout and character of medieval Brighton. The townspeople continued to rely on fishing for their prosperity, and in the 1580s Brighton was one of the most important south-coast fishing ports, with 80 vessels, 400 fishermen and about 10,000 nets. There was always tension between the fishermen and the landsmen. In the 16th century the cost of defending the town fell mainly to the fishermen, who petitioned the Privy Council to spread the expense. As a result 'The Booke of Auncient Customs' was drawn up, detailing the organisation and financing of the local fishing industry, and a local government body was created – 'The Twelve' (8 fishermen and 4 landsmen) to assist in

◄ **1** *George IV by Sir Francis Chantrey (a copy in bronze of the marble statue at Windsor), erected on the Steine in 1828, the cost of £3000 being defrayed by public subscription. In 1922 the statue was moved to its present site by the North Gate of the Pavilion to make way for the War Memorial. George IV, who is inextricably linked with Brighton's rise to fame as a fashionable resort, ruled Britain as Regent from 1811 and became King in 1820, after one of the most magnificent and extravagant coronations ever seen.*

the enforcement of law and order, and to supervise repairs both to the church and to the town's defences. But the fishing industry began to decline in the 17th century, as local boats suffered harassment from foreign vessels and increasing competition from other British fishing fleets jealously guarding what they saw as their rights.

In 1657 occurred one of the most famous episodes in Brighton's early history, the escape of the future Charles II after his defeat by Parliamentary forces at the Battle of Worcester. Many stories have grown up around this event. Apparently Charles was brought here by Colonel Gounter, a local Royalist landowner, and Francis Mancell, a merchant from Chichester, who had persuaded a local shipowner, Captain Nicholas Tettersal, to carry 'two friends' of theirs – supposedly fleeing the country because of their involvement in a duel – to France for the sum of £50. The party spent the night at the now demolished George Inn, thought to have stood on the western side of West St – then a lonely part of the town, and so highly suitable. The innkeeper and Tettersal both recognised Charles, and it took much persuasion, and more money, before he was able to sail from the nearby port of Shoreham for Fécamp, in Normandy; only two hours later troops arrived in Brighton to search for him. After the Restoration of the monarchy in 1660, Tettersal was rewarded with a pension and made High Constable of Brighton, in which role he mounted a thorough and vindictive persecution of local Quakers and other Nonconformists.

In the 17th and 18th centuries the sea, ever a threat to the town, encroached even further inland, the worst damage being done in two terrible storms. The severity of the first, in 1703, led Daniel Defoe to write a treatise on storms which describes how in Brighton 'the violence of the wind stript a great many houses, turn'd up the leads off the church, overthrew two windmills . . . the town in general looking as if it had been bombarded'. In 1705 the lower town was totally destroyed, all its houses being buried under a mound of shingle, and the sea began to threaten the upper town. The only solution was to build wooden groynes which would cause an accumulation of protective shingle on the beach, but the population of Brighton was too impoverished to pay for them; so permission was granted for an appeal for funds to be made in churches and chapels throughout the county. The steadily decreasing population reached its nadir of around 1000 in 1740, and those who did live in Brighton were so poor that three-quarters of all houses were exempt from rates. There seemed a real possibility that the town might fall a victim to the sea when, by an ironic twist of fate, it was the fact that it was situated by the sea that led to Brighton's revival and transformation.

The first record of sea-bathing at Brighton comes from a letter of the Rev. William Clarke, who spent the summer of 1736 here with his family: 'my morning business is bathing in the sea . . .', he wrote to a friend. Nearly 20 years elapsed, however, before many people practised this novelty or, indeed, even visited the impoverished town. Then in 1750 Dr Richard Russell, from nearby Lewes, published *De Tabe Glandulari Sive De Usu Aquae Marinae In Morbis Glandularum Dissertio*. In this book he strongly advocated both swimming in and drinking sea water as a cure for various diseases, especially those affecting the glands. The medical profession was impressed (though the ideas were not entirely new), and when an English translation appeared, Russell's 'cure' became famous. Brighton being the nearest seaside town to Lewes, it was the destination of Dr Russell's patients.

► *2 St Nicholas' church, much restored in 1853, retains its 14th-century nave, chancel arch and tower. The interior contains several interesting memorials, including one to the Duke of Wellington, who went to school in Brighton. The chief pride of the church is its 12th-century font, an exquisitely carved piece of Caen stone, which possibly came from the Cluniac priory at Lewes to which Brighton was attached; this would account for the high quality of the work. The scenes depicted on it are the Last Supper, the Baptism of Christ, and episodes from the life of St Nicholas, one of them a delightful representation of the Saint in a boat, saving the lives of pilgrims by thwarting the approaches of the devil. In the churchyard are memorials to several well-known local figures, including Amon Wilds (see p. 17), Nicholas Tettersal (see p. 8), Phoebe Hassell (see p. 14) and Martha Gunn. Brighton has some splendid Victorian churches too, notably St Michael's, Victoria Road, with windows by Rossetti and Morris, and the grandly proportioned St Bartholomew's, Ann St.*

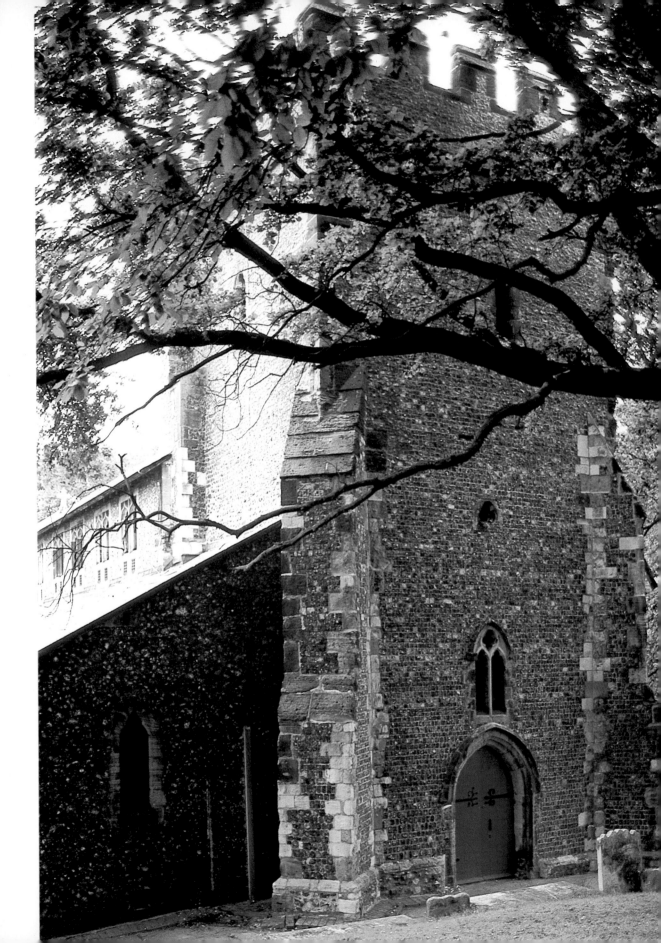

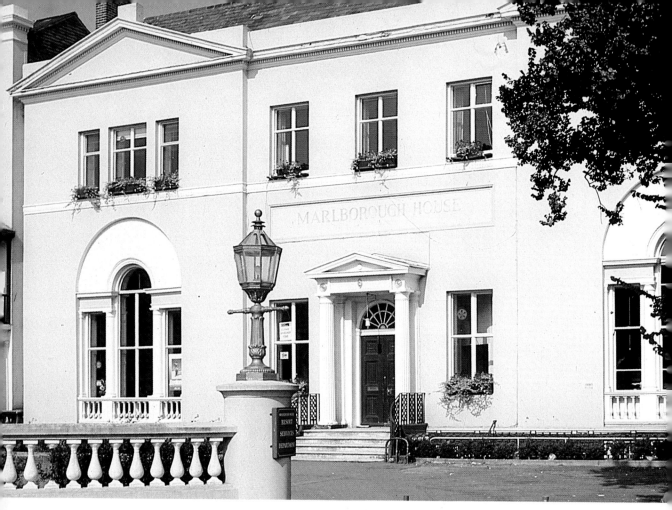

Sea-bathing can hardly have been pleasurable when it was done, as most doctors recommended, early in the day during the winter; the novelist Fanny Burney, in describing her 'dip at dawn' on a November morning as 'cold but pleasant', explained that 'I have bathed so often as to lose my dread of the operation'. In those days very few people could actually swim, so they were always attended by a 'bather' or 'dipper', who would hold them and plunge them into the water from the steps of a bathing machine. Many of these attendants became well-known local figures, including 'Smoaker' Miles, the Prince Regent's bather, and Martha Gunn. Six years before his death in 1759, Russell moved to Brighton; he had a house built at the south end of the Steine, where the Royal Albion Hotel now stands. His successors included Dr Anthony Relhan, who wrote a tract extolling Brighton's healthy climate, and Dr Awister, whose prescriptions included drinking a mixture of sea water and milk, and who had hot and cold sea water baths built in Pool Valley for those who could not face the rigours of the sea itself. It was during their time that Brighton began to emerge as a fashionable watering place, and soon both patients and ordinary visitors began to flock to the town in ever-increasing numbers. Its rising popularity was helped by its position as the south-coast town most accessible from London – though in the 1750s, reaching it by carrier's wagon could take two days. By the 1820s express coaches were accomplishing the journey in 5¼ hours.

Initially there was little for the visitors to do, and few places for them to stay

▲ 3 *Marlborough House (1769), architecturally one of Brighton's most important houses, was built by Samuel Shergold, proprietor of the Castle Hotel. The next owner, the Duke of Marlborough, sold it (1786) to William Hamilton, who employed Robert Adam to redesign it. The drawing room has a Sicilian marble fireplace and there is a charming octagonal dining room; the house is one of the few surviving examples of Adam's work on a small domestic scale.*

except small lodging houses owned by fishermen. The only hotels of any consequence were the Castle (now demolished) and the Old Ship, and both were quick to capitalise on the town's new popularity. By the 1760s both had Assembly Rooms, where balls and card parties were held under the auspices of the Master of Ceremonies appointed to organise the social life of the town during the fashionable season (June–September). The first and most famous Master of Ceremonies was Captain Wade, who also held the same position in Bath for several years. The visitors' pattern of life followed that of the spas of Bath and Tunbridge Wells. Apart from an early morning dip, a typical day's activities might include a public breakfast, a promenade along the Steine, and a visit to the library. This last was a very important aspect of Brighton life, corresponding socially to the Pump Rooms of the spas. The first libraries included Thomas' and Baker's; here subscribers would meet to read the papers, gossip, and – perhaps most important – study the lists of new arrivals in a book kept up to date by the Master of Ceremonies. The first permanent theatre was built in North St in 1774, the present Theatre Royal being erected in New Road in 1807. For the more energetic visitor, there was hunting on the Downs, or racing: the first organised race meeting took place in 1783, and the subsequent annual meetings were often attended by the Prince Regent. These and many other attractions drew all fashionable and literary society. The Thrale family had a house built in West St (now the site of Sherry's Dance Hall), and their visitors, besides Fanny Burney, included Dr Johnson – who however declared the place 'so truly desolate, that if one had a mind to hang oneself for desperation at being obliged to live there, it would be difficult to find a tree on which to fasten the rope'. The threat of war against France led to the establishment of a military camp just outside the town in 1793, adding to Brighton's liveliness and giving the feather-brained Lydia in Jane Austen's *Pride and Prejudice* cause to

► **4** *A model of a hog boat in Brighton Museum. 'Hoggies', used by mackerel fishermen, were developed to suit the conditions of the Brighton coastline in a form that could be easily launched off the shingle beach. Having a great deal of beam in proportion to their length, they were very stable even in rough seas. Hoggies were used in Brighton until the end of the 19th century, when the last one was burned on the beach at a 5th November bonfire.*

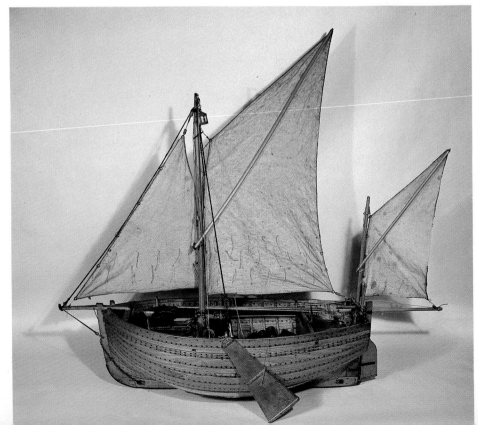

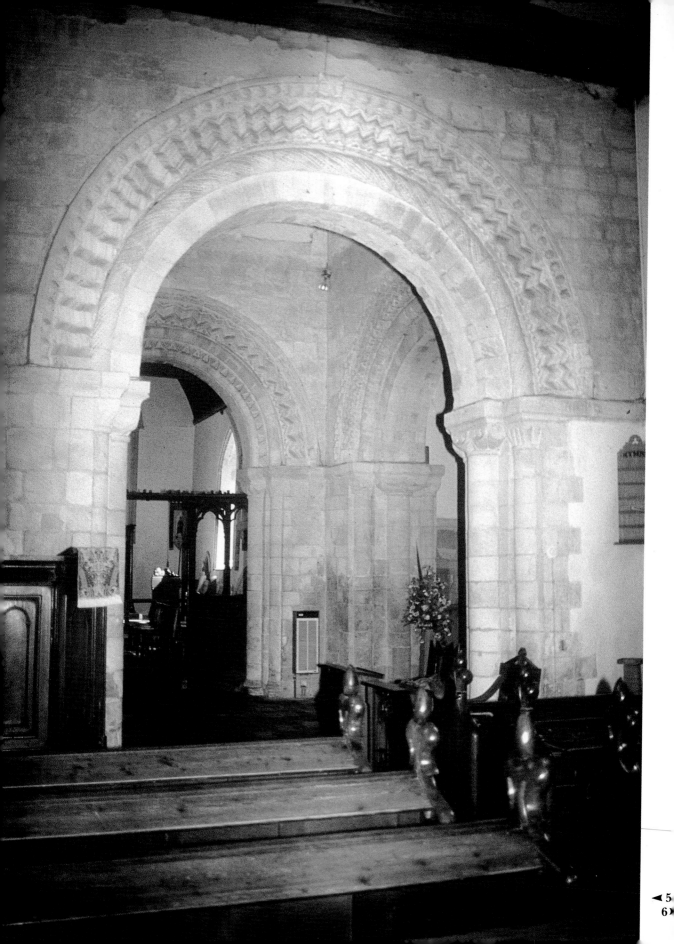

◄ 5
6►

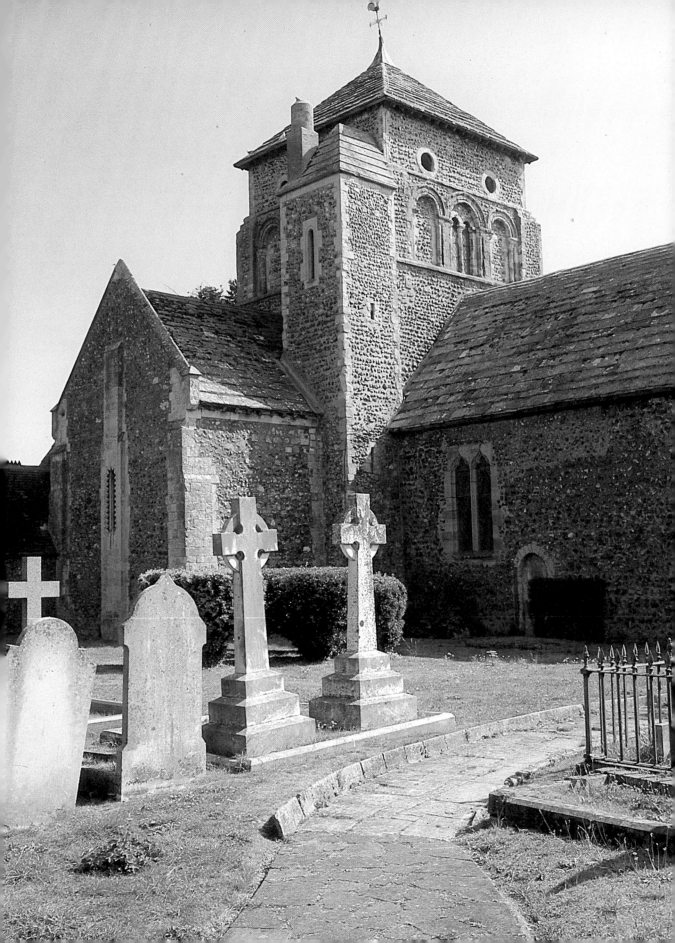

believe that 'a visit to Brighton comprised every possibility of earthly happiness', not least because 'that is the place to get husbands'.

Soon the Royal family was attracted to Brighton; it was to visit his uncle the Duke of Cumberland that the 21-year-old Prince of Wales first came here on 7 September 1783 – a cause for great local celebration and a tremendous welcome (marred by the death of a gunner firing the Royal Salute). It has been suggested that the Prince came to try sea-bathing as a cure for swollen neck glands. Whatever the reason, he was enchanted by the place, and his visits became a more or less annual event. Brighton's future prosperity was thus assured as it was now the semi-permanent residence of the heir apparent. The Prince was always popular locally, whatever feelings were about him elsewhere; his generosity to Brighton causes and people, such as the celebrated Phoebe Hassell, to whom he paid a weekly pension of half a guinea, was well known and appreciated. (Phoebe Hassell, who lived to be 108, had in her youth disguised herself as a boy and joined the British Army to be near her soldier lover, who had been posted to the West Indies. It was only after 17 years, when he was wounded, that she revealed her still undetected secret to the regimental Colonel's wife.) The Prince's birthdays were always marked in Brighton with bell-ringing, all kinds of races just outside the town, the roasting of an ox for the townspeople and a ball in the evening when the whole town was illuminated. For the Prince, Brighton provided the setting in which he could fully enjoy his new-found freedom from his parents and from the stuffy ways of the court at Windsor. His affairs with women were many and much talked about, none more so than his relationship with Mrs Maria Fitzherbert, a twice-widowed Roman Catholic, whom he secretly (and illegally) married in 1785. At Brighton they spent many of their happiest days, though always maintaining separate establishments.

Having decided that he wanted a permanent base here, the Prince commissioned the architect Henry Holland to design a residence for him. The Marine Pavilion, completed within 4 months in 1787, was a simple classical building in the Palladian style, with a central rotunda and bow-fronted wings to north and south. (It still forms the nucleus of the Pavilion, hidden by later building.) The Prince occupied rooms on the upper floor of the south wing, and reputedly had a reflecting glass fitted in his bedroom so that he could watch the comings and goings on the Steine while lying in bed. He was not long content with his new home, and additions and alterations were continually made, inside and out. In the 1800s the interior began to be refurbished in striking and fanciful Chinese style by Frederick Crace & Sons; in 1805 the great domed stables in Indian style (designed by William Porden) were erected (17), provoking the comment that the Prince's horses were better housed than he was himself. The style of the stables gave the Prince ideas for dramatic alterations to his Pavilion, and by 1815 he had sufficient resources. Of several architects who submitted plans John Nash was chosen to effect the transformation. By 1822 the building was in its present-day form. It contains a great mixture of styles, but the Indian inspiration clearly dominates; it is a building without parallel in this country, and contemporary reaction to it was at best mixed. William Hazlitt thought it looked 'like a collection of stone pumpkins and pepper boxes . . . anything more fantastical with a greater dearth of invention was never seen'. Several commented on the similarity with the Kremlin, in Moscow. The King (as he had now become) seemed pleased enough with his new home, though not with the

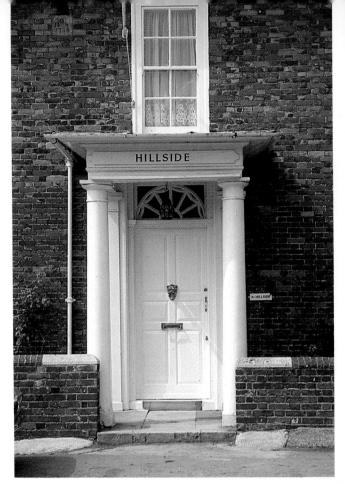

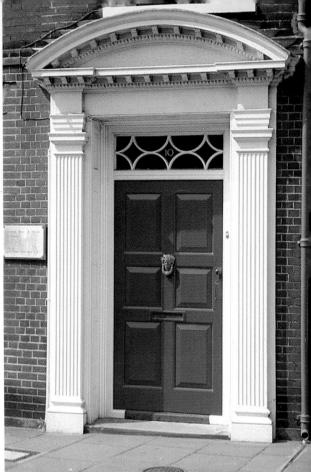

**▲7**                                               **8▼**

*Brighton and its surroundings offer constant delights to the lover of 18th-century and Regency architecture, from the grand sweeps of the crescents to varied details like the doorways shown here.* **7** (above left): *Hillside is a handsome red brick Queen Anne house, architecturally the finest in the charming village of Rottingdean, a few miles east of Brighton. Its doorway is surrounded by a porch with Tuscan columns. In the years before World War I Hillside was leased by the actor-manager Herbert Beerbohm Tree, who entertained the leading figures of society, including Lady Diana Manners, the future Lady Diana Cooper.* **8** (above right): *10, Prince Albert St, also of red brick, is one of the few really spacious 18th-century houses in Brighton. The doorway is an excellent example of modern reconstruction, as is the whole of the ground floor.* **9** (right): *68, Ship St, like most of the houses in this street, also dates from the 18th century.*

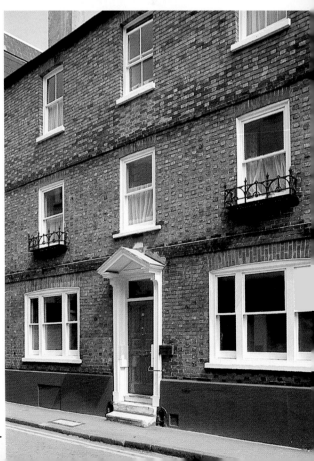

**9►**

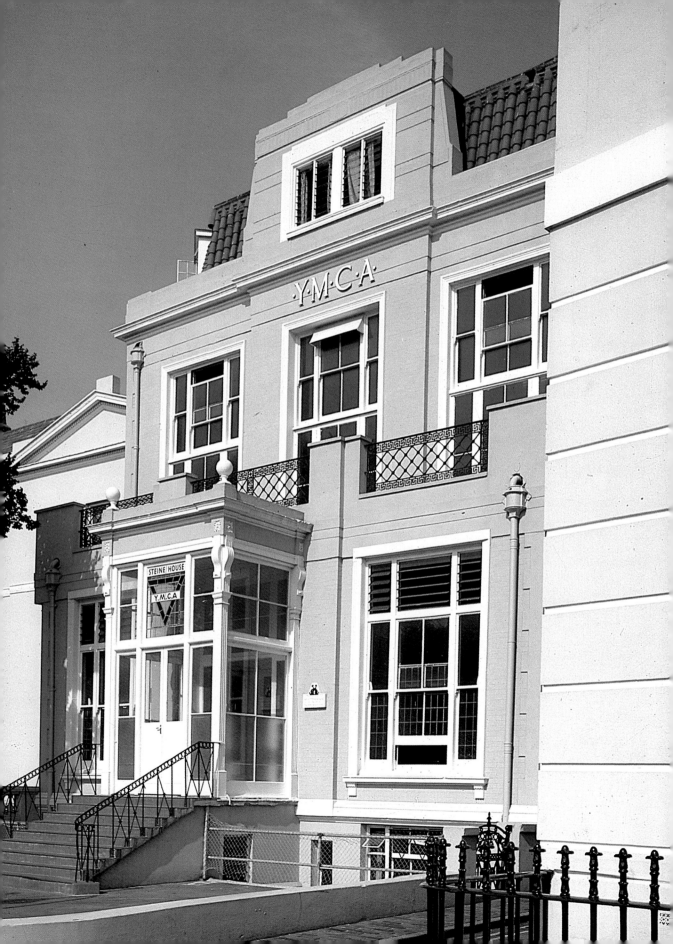

cost of it (Nash had never presented an estimate), but in fact for the last few years of his life he spent much less time than formerly at Brighton. He always had a reputation for fast living and keeping unsuitable company, and inevitably stories of wild goings-on at the Pavilion began to circulate; but what the majority of eyewitnesses seemed to remark about an evening spent there was the intense heat of the rooms. Certainly Mrs Fitzherbert had a sobering influence on the Prince, but though he is said to have declared that she was the 'wife of his heart and soul' he twice abandoned her: in 1795, to marry Caroline of Brunswick, and again in 1811. She kept her house in Brighton, where she remained a popular figure, 'treated as a Queen', as the Whig politician Thomas Creevey remarked, 'at least of Brighton'. William IV was kind to her and offered to make her a Duchess. This she refused, but she did consent to her servants' wearing Royal livery. She died in 1837. Her monument in the Roman Catholic church of St John the Baptist, Bristol Road, shows her wearing the three wedding rings of her three marriages.

In 1791 the *Sussex Weekly Advertiser* declared, 'so great has been the increase of Company within these last few days at Brighton that there is not now a house on the Steine or on the Bank to be let', and the town spread as the annual number of visitors increased. Although Brighton is often described as a 'Regency' town, most building took place not during the Regency era but in the decade 1820–30, when the number of houses almost doubled. Much of this new building was the collaborative work of the local builder-architect Amon Wilds (born 1762) and C. A. Busby (1799–1834), who came to Brighton from a successful career in London and America. One of their first major projects was Thomas Read Kemp's grandiose scheme of Kemp Town (see **53**); other work included Brunswick Town (**45**) and much of Marine Parade (**52**). Meanwhile Amon Wilds' son, A. H. Wilds, working mainly on his own, designed much of Park Crescent, Western Terrace, and Montpelier Crescent (**47**). The architect of another important building dating from this period, St Peter's church (1824–8), was Charles Barry, who later designed the Houses of Parliament. St Peter's is one of the finest churches of the early Gothic revival. Originally built as a chapel of ease for St Nicholas', it became Brighton parish church in 1873.

The death of George IV in 1830 did little to diminish the popularity of the town. His successor William IV regularly stayed at the Pavilion with his wife Queen Adelaide, and they made additions to it in the form of the South Lodge, 'Queen Adelaide's Stables' in Church St (converted later into the present Art Gallery and Museum), and the North Lodge and Gate. One of William's favourite occupations was strolling up and down the newly erected Chain Pier, where he would stop to converse with some of his rather bemused subjects, and buy sweets for the children who followed him around. The Chain Pier (1823) was the first pier in Britain. Built as a landing place for the packet boats from France, it soon proved popular as a promenade for visitors. It was designed by Samuel Brown on the same principles as a suspension bridge, and stretched out to sea for 1134 ft. In December 1896, only 2 months after it had been declared unsafe and closed to the public, it was completely destroyed by a violent storm.

Queen Victoria and Prince Albert visited the Pavilion in their turn, but with little enthusiasm – partly because, as Victoria wrote to her aunt, 'the people are very indiscreet and troublesome here really, which makes the place quite a prison'. In February 1845 the Royal family left Brighton for the last time, and in future spent their holidays at Osborne House, on the Isle of Wight. Gradually all the Pavilion's furniture and fittings were removed to Windsor and Buckingham Palace, and it seemed likely that the building would be demolished. But the townspeople had grown attached to this odd structure in their midst, and opposed any such move. Eventually the local governing body, the Town Commissioners, acquired the Royal Pavilion for Brighton in 1850 for £50,000, a tiny fraction of what it had cost George IV. At once repairs and redecorations were effected, and in January 1851 a ball attended by 1400 people was held to celebrate the formal opening of the interior. The building was used for similar functions, as well as business meetings, concerts and lectures, for the next 100 years. Visitors continued to throng to Brighton, among them many of the famous writers and artists of the day: Thackeray, Dickens, who wrote much of *Dombey and Son* and *Bleak House* here, and Constable, who spent several summers here with his family between 1824 and 1839. He made a number of oil sketches of the coast and was evidently fascinated by the Chain Pier, which appears in *The Marine Parade and Chain Pier* (now in the Tate Gallery, London).

The railway between London and Brighton opened in September 1841, causing great local excitement and celebration. The first excursion train ran from London at Easter 1844, carrying hundreds of day trippers to the seaside in about 4½ hours. This was the start of the tourist phenomenon that reached its height in the 1860s, when the Whit Monday of 1862 saw about 130,000 visitors descend on Brighton – a not entirely welcome development. Many felt that the trippers did the town little good, sitting on the beach for most of the day and spending what little money they had on drink. But a new era was clearly dawning. Brighton was no longer a select watering place, but a seaside town where people came to enjoy themselves. Soon all manner of amusements were

▼ 11 *The beach first thing in the morning, with only a few hardy swimmers taking an early dip. Although it is mainly shingle, this 7-mile beach has always been one of the main attractions of Brighton and Hove, and on sunny days it quickly fills up with people of all ages, building sand castles, paddling, taking boats out, swimming, water-skiing, windsurfing, or just sitting in deck chairs sunbathing.*

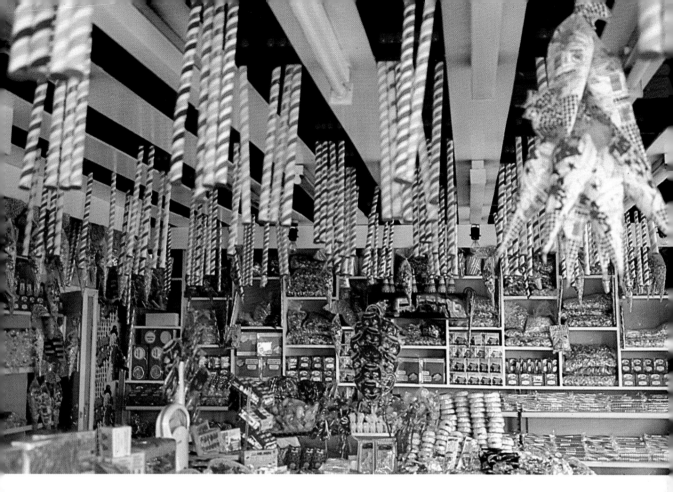

catering for them: the West Pier (1866); the Palace Pier (1899), replacing the Chain Pier; the highly popular Aquarium (opened 1872); and Volk's Railway. This was the first (1883) regular electric train service in Britain, albeit a short one – originally along the shore between the Aquarium and the Chain Pier. It was the brainchild of Magnus Volk, a Brighton man, who was also the first person to install domestic electric light and a telephone system in the town. He achieved his great aim of extending his railway to the nearby village of Rotting-dean in 1896; so that the train could run whatever the state of the tide, it was mounted on stilts 24 ft high, earning it the name of 'Daddy Long Legs'. Tourists loved it, but eventually this part of the line had to close, giving way to the construction of groynes to prevent cliff erosion. The railway still operates along the front (Palace Pier to Black Rock Pool), from April to September.

In Victorian times as now, the beach was the main attraction – though most people sat on it fully clothed, there being no such thing as swimwear, and bathing machines being expensive and over-subscribed (bathing machines continued in use until Edwardian times). A distinction developed between the noisy, crowded centre of the town, around the Chain and later the Palace Pier, where the trippers tended to congregate, and the more refined western end of the town, where the fashionable hotels were situated; some of the most particular visitors moved even further west into Hove, which in the 1890s established itself as a suburb for the affluent retired. After a period of depression in the first years of the 20th century, when the upper classes virtually deserted Brighton, the regular visits of Edward VII made the town fashionable again. In

1908 the luxury train The Southern Belle started to run between London and Brighton, and in September 1910 the list of visitors included 5 Dukes, 4 Duchesses, 1 Marquis, 23 Earls, 33 Barons and all the principal members of the Cabinet. The advent of the motor car also boosted the town's fortunes, Brighton being a good distance for a day trip from London. The trials and tribulations of these early vehicles are commemorated in the annual veteran car run, and were immortalised in the film *Genevieve*.

During World War I Brighton became a haven from the air raids on London, and for the wounded: at George V's suggestion the Pavilion was used as a hospital for Indian soldiers, and over 4000 had been treated there by April 1916. The commemorative South Gate of the Pavilion was erected as the gift of the Indian people in 1921. During World War II the threat of invasion was once again very real; the beaches were mined and wired off, the piers were blown up in the middle, and visitors were barred from the town, which wore a strange deserted air. Between the wars Brighton gained rather an unpleasant reputation as the centre of ruthless, underworld gangs (luridly portrayed in Graham Greene's *Brighton Rock*), which culminated at a Lewes race meeting in 1936, when the gangs were finally beaten after a fight between the police and the notorious Hoxton Mob. Violence returned to Brighton in the 1960s, this time on the beaches, with the seemingly ritual Bank Holiday clashes between the rival gangs of 'Mods' and 'Rockers' – now a thing of the past.

Brighton in the 20th century has also faced the conflict, common to many historic towns, between preservation and progress. Much of the building before 1945 was haphazard, and it was to oppose such developments as Embassy Court, a towering block of flats right next to Brunswick Terrace, and to ensure

▼ **13** *Sussex University: the Engineering and Applied Sciences building. The 200-acre campus, near the village of Falmer, is planned as a series of related zones linked by footpaths, with buildings grouped round informal courtyards – sciences to the east and arts and social sciences to the west. The distinctive architecture is unified by the use of local materials, especially a russet brick, and is sensitively accommodated to its beautiful parkland setting in the South Downs. Sir Basil Spence was the architect of the first buildings and of much of the layout.*

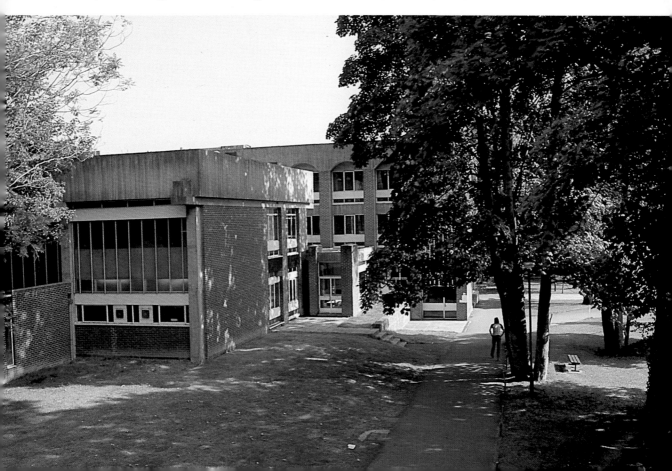

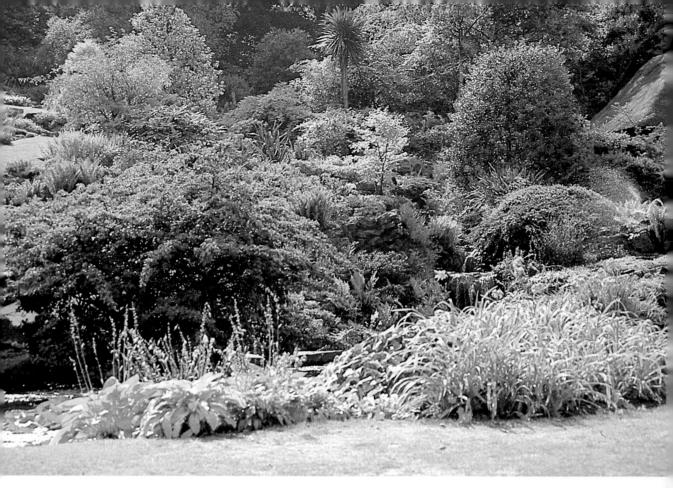

**▲ 14** *Preston Rock Gardens. Brighton is justly proud of its fine municipal parks and gardens, which cover 3000 acres. These beautifully tended rock gardens, their subtle colours contrasting with the bright flowerbeds on the opposite side of the London Road, are in Preston, to the north of the town. Now totally engulfed by Brighton, this was once a separate village called Prestetone, meaning a priest's holding, and belonged to the Bishopric of Chichester.*

the preservation of Brighton's historic buildings, that the Regency Society was formed in 1945. Even the Pavilion was once threatened with demolition, but restoration under the energetic guidance of successive Keepers, helped by the permanent loan by the Royal family of much of the original furniture, has returned it to its former glory and made it Brighton's greatest architectural attraction. The £10 million refurbishment is now complete (**15, 18**). More than any other seaside town Brighton has coped with the competition to its tourist trade offered by cheap continental travel, creating new attractions (see p. 56) and developing in other areas. It has become the home of many London commuters, among them several well-known actors and actresses including, at one time, Laurence Olivier and Joan Plowright. The University of Sussex, granted its charter in 1961, is one of the major employers in the county. Besides being the first of Britain's post-war universities, it pioneered the adoption in England of broadly based undergraduate courses, in which students work within different schools – European, Afro-Asian or American – rather than single subjects. In 1989 there were 5300 students, many of them renting rooms in Brighton formerly taken by holidaymakers and doing much valuable voluntary community work. The excellent programmes of the University's Gardner Arts Centre, open to all, greatly enrich the cultural life of the area. The proliferation of language schools in the 1970s also served to diversify and strengthen the local economy. Through the centuries Brighton has adapted well, if sometimes by accident, to new challenges, while retaining its unique charm. It remains what Horace Smith so rightly dubbed it, 'the Queen of Watering Places'.

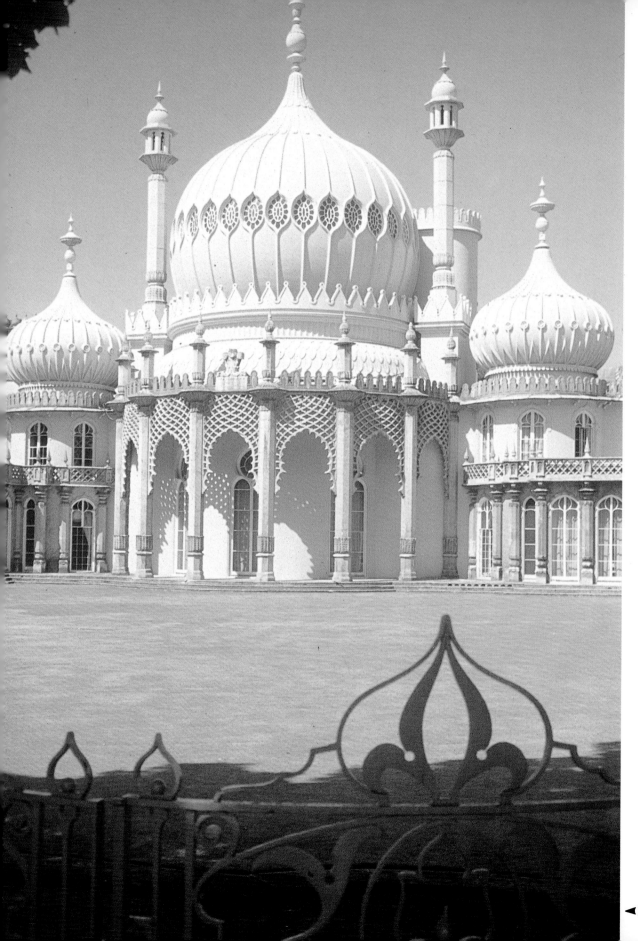

# A Tour of the Centre

English interest in India and its culture, which had been growing since the early 17th century, was stimulated from 1795 by the publication of Thomas Daniell's series of views, *Oriental Scenery*. This showed the English the great beauty of Mughal Indian buildings, which provided the dominant inspiration for Nash's remodelling of the Prince Regent's Pavilion in 1815. (A notable earlier attempt to emulate the Indian style, Sezincote (1805), near Moreton-in-Marsh, Gloucestershire, was in part Thomas Daniell's creation and may have influenced the Prince, as he was a visitor there.) The Pavilion's entire eastern front, along the Steine (**15**), was clothed with an oriental colonnade, the columns being linked with Indian 'jalis' of pierced stone latticework; this and the continuous cornice of the Indian battlements give the building a sense of unity. The west front is perhaps less dramatically lovely, but has its own charm with its irregular outline. The large central Indian dome and the pair of smaller ones flanking it have been the subject of many jibes, but their squat form is offset by the minarets – some decorative, some disguised chimneys – which fill up every spare space on the roof. The last part of the Pavilion to be completed, the north front, housed the King's apartments and accommodation for visitors; it has a very neat outline with balconies and an Indian colonnade. The Pavilion was built of Bath stone and brick covered with stucco. Nash's innovative use of the new medium of cast-iron for the internal support of elaborate stonework has over the years caused problems, in that the iron rusts and corrodes the stone, which is now undergoing repair and conservation.

The colourful Pavilion Gardens (**16**) provide the opportunity to relax in tranquil surroundings only a few yards from the town centre and enjoy such traditional seaside entertainments as brass band concerts and, occasionally, Punch and Judy shows. There were pleasure gardens here in the late 18th century, the Brighthelmston Pleasure Grove, a venue for public breakfasts, concerts, races and firework displays.

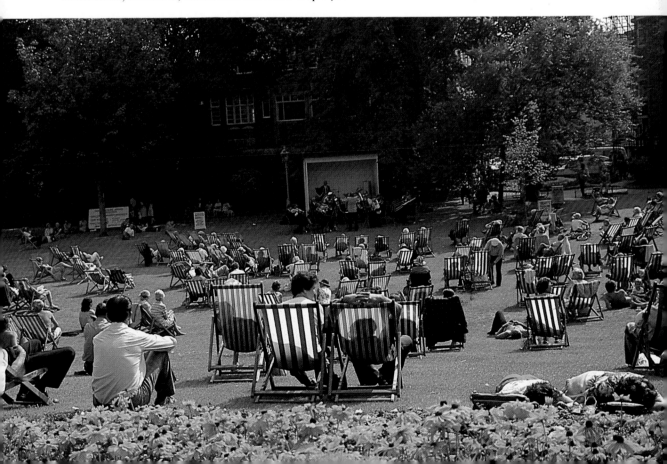

The Dome (**17**), built 1803–5, formerly the Prince Regent's riding stables, takes its name from its enormous central cupola. This measures 85 ft across and 65 ft in height, and represents a remarkable engineering feat for its day: indeed at the time it was widely believed that the whole building would collapse. The architect, William Porden, drew his inspiration from the Cornmarket in Paris and the Great Mosque in Delhi. Forty horses were housed in stalls in a great circle, with a pool and fountain for watering them in the centre; in a balcony were harness rooms and accommodation for grooms and coachmen. Nowadays the Dome is used for conferences and concerts. It seats over 2000. The Riding House (10,000 sq ft), behind the Dome, built at the same time for the Prince to exercise his horses, became the Corn Exchange in the late 19th century and is now an exhibition hall.

The Banqueting Room (**18**), the climax of the Pavilion's interior transformation in thoroughgoing Chinoiserie, was chiefly designed by Robert Jones. Its rich colour and opulence, especially by contrast with the approach from a low and rather dark corridor, is spectacular. The ceiling, a 45-ft dome, is painted a vivid blue, against which lies the foliage of a plantain tree, partly modelled in copper. From this hangs a gilt dragon which carries a huge gasolier, 30 ft high and a ton in weight, with more dragons radiating from it. (In William IV's reign the gasolier was taken down after Queen Adelaide had a dream about it crashing to the ground.) In each corner of the room smaller gasoliers hang from the Fum, a legendary bird of Chinese mythology, one of the four symbolic figures which kept guard over the Empire. The walls are painted with 'Chinese scenes', framed in red and yellow blind fret; the window draperies were deep crimson satin tinged with gold; and the canopied ceilings at either end of the room were decorated in gold with birds, flowers and dragons hanging from the roof.

▼ **17 18**

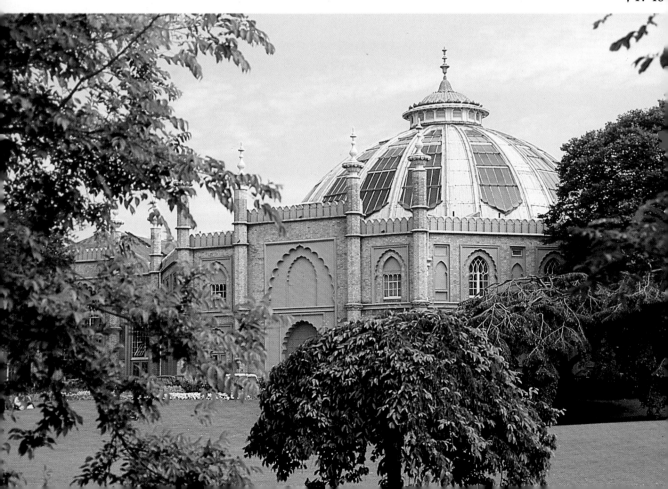

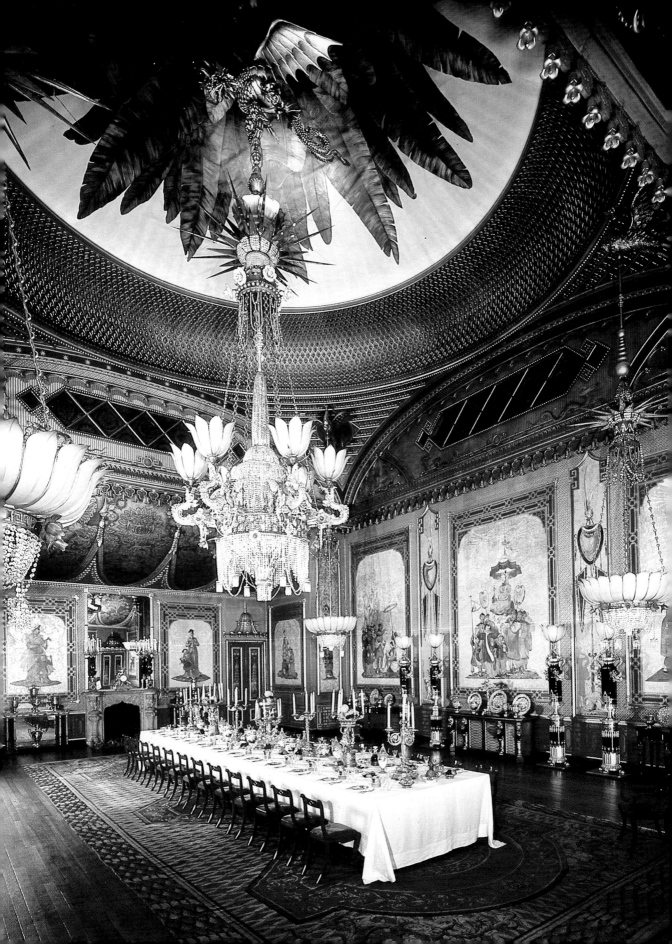

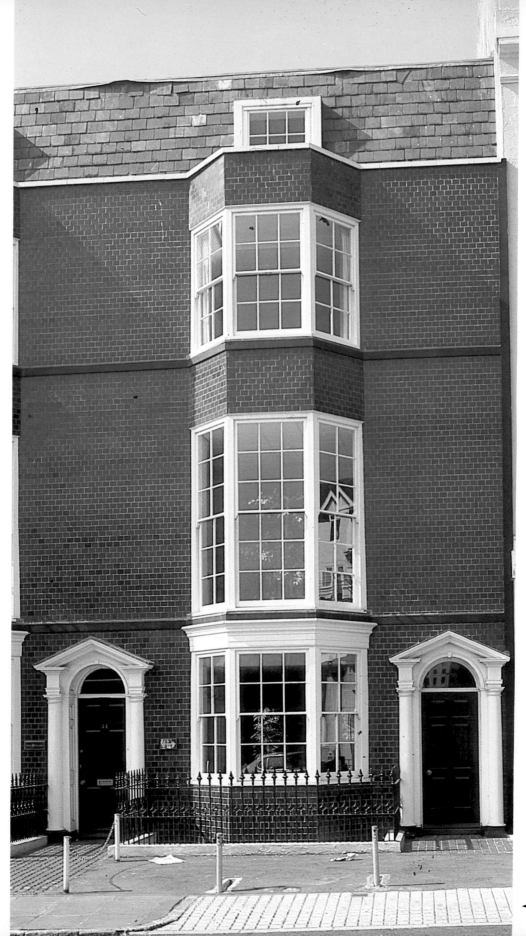

44–45, Old Steine (**19**), recently refurbished as offices, are among the few late-18th-century houses in the Steine to survive with little alteration. They are fronted with the black 'mathematical' tiles characteristic of many houses in Brighton. These look like shiny black bricks, but are in fact small facing tiles hung on a wooden frame, and are used on seaside houses because they resist sea spray and harsh winds much better than ordinary bricks and tiles.

The Steine (*steine* is Scandinavian for a stone), formerly common land where fishermen dried their nets and beached their boats during storms, became the fashionable promenade in the 18th century. Its enclosure in the 19th century caused angry demonstrations by the fishermen, who felt they were being deprived of their ancient rights. As the town spread east and west during succeeding years the Steine lost some of its identity as Brighton's focal point, but despite heavy traffic it retains, with its shady walks and colourful flowerbeds, an atmosphere of genteel urban leisure. Steine Gardens (**20**) are dominated by the sparkling fountain designed by A. H. Wilds, who was responsible for much of Brighton's early-19th-century architecture. The lower base of its elaborate structure rests on the entwined figures of three dolphins, which also form part of the coat of arms of the Borough of Brighton.

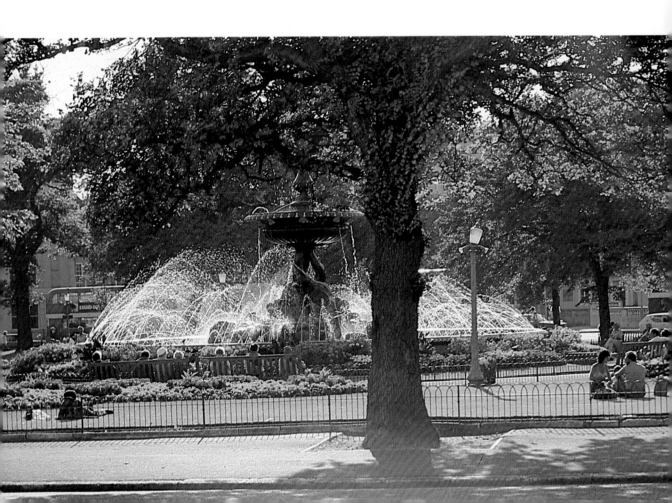

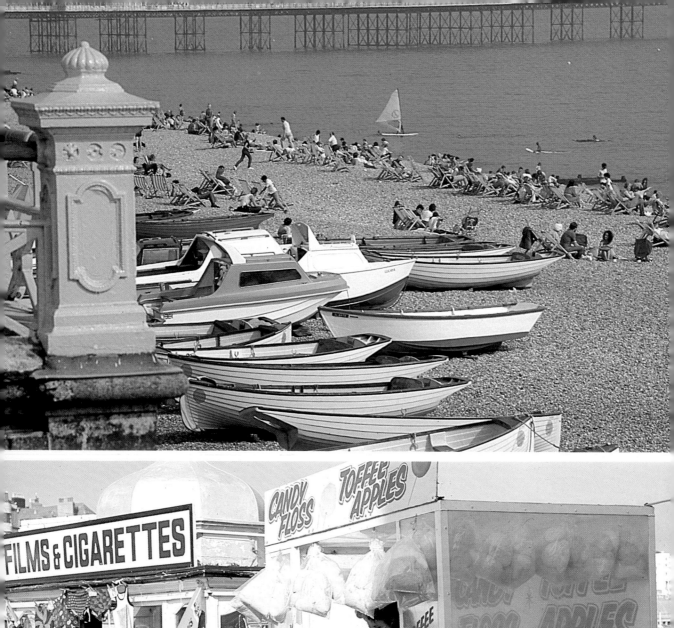
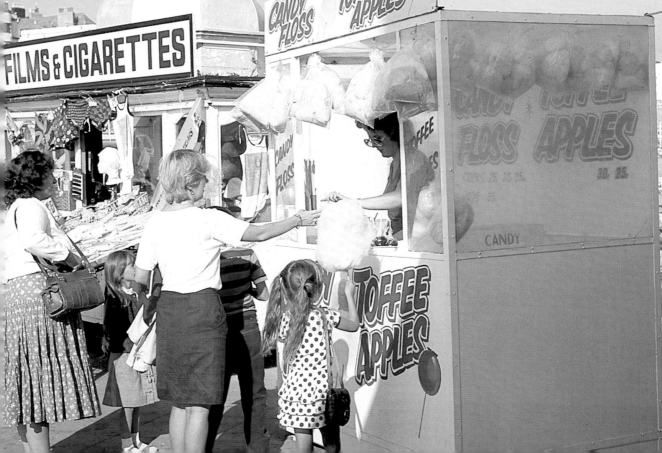

The Palace Pier was designed to replace the old Chain Pier, which the new West Pier had overtaken as a fashionable attraction. Although building started in 1891, it was not complete until 1899, by which time the Chain Pier had been destroyed by a storm (1896). The new pier was an immediate success with visitors, and has remained so, being thought by many to be the finest ever built. Its oriental domes and delicate filigree-work arches clearly show the influence of the Pavilion on its design. Initially every arch and roof-line was illuminated by electric lights, but after World War II (during which the pier was partly destroyed as a defensive measure) not all of these were replaced. The pierhead platform, with an ornate theatre, was added in 1901 and improved in 1911, when a bandstand and winter garden (now the Palace of Fun) were also constructed. The Palace Pier Repertory Company presented a wide and varied programme until lack of support forced it to disband in 1964. The theatre now houses the National Museum of Penny Slot Machines, and is full of the gadgets that delighted people at the turn of the century; for one old penny (available at the Museum) you can see 'Two Lovely Ladies' or 'What The Butler Didn't See'. The pier has always offered promenaders a wide variety of amusements and today you can still sample many traditional seaside delights here – buy whelks and mussels, candy floss, sticks of rock and all sorts of souvenirs, have your palm read by a clairvoyant, have your photograph taken with a marmoset, catch a fish, take a ride on the ghost train, or just enjoy a walk in the bracing sea air.

**21**: The pier from the beach to the west; **22**: the entrance – the original entrance of three arches in delicate ironwork was replaced in 1930 by the present entrance and clock-tower, when the Aquarium was rebuilt and the sea road widened; **23**: strolling down the west side of the pier. OVERLEAF: **24**: the Palace of Fun; **25**: the view from the end of the pier, east toward Kemp Town and Black Rock; **26**: looking west towards the West Pier; **27**: the end of the day, cleaners in the tea room.

23▼

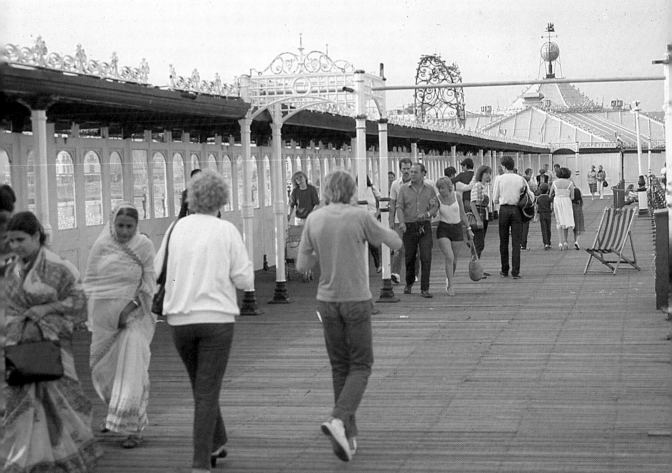

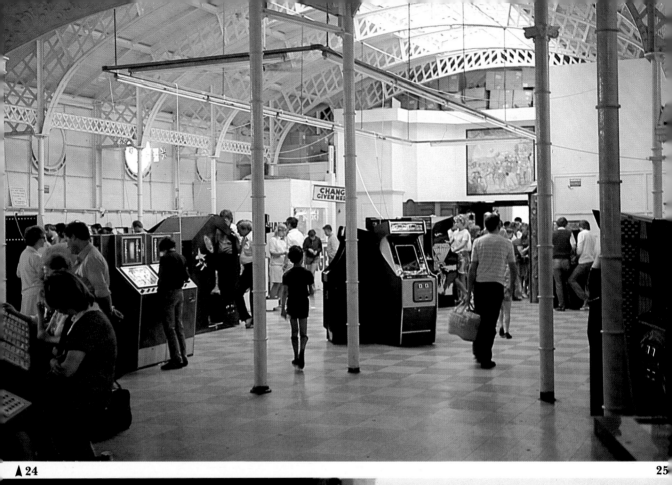

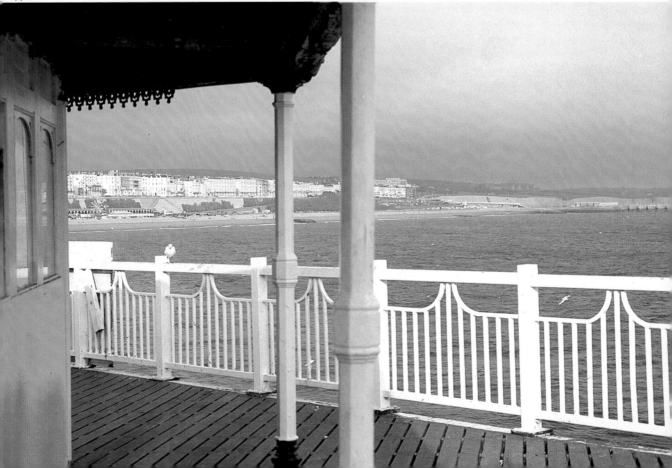

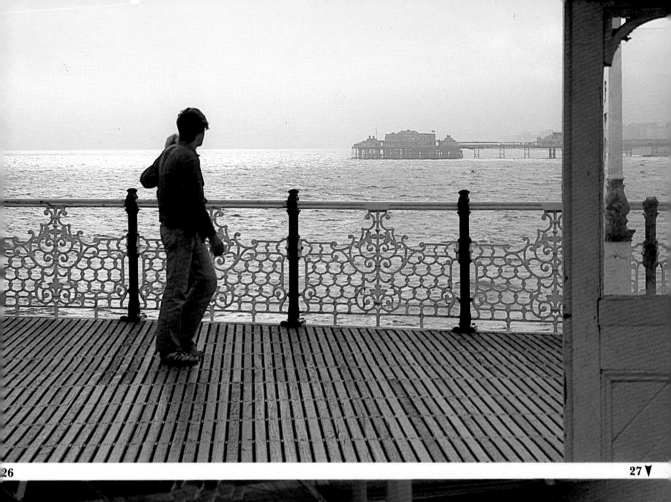

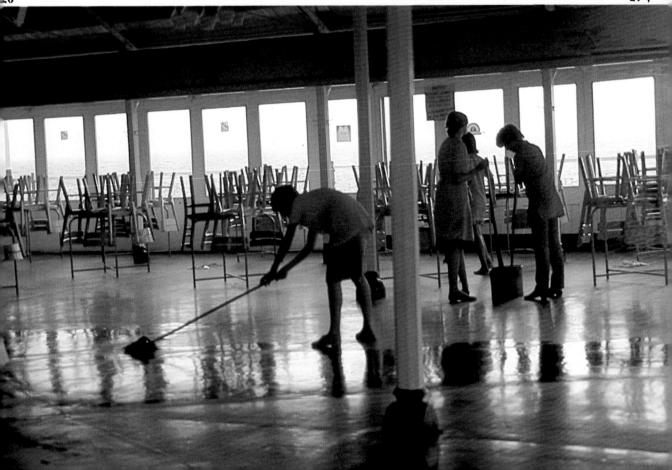

The Lanes, the centre of medieval Brighton, were formerly a series of ill-lit narrow alleyways, known locally as twittens. Now they are lively and bustling, one of the most visited parts of Brighton. The narrow streets with overhanging upper stories, full of antique shops, jewellers, boutiques and craft stores, give a feeling of the old town, though most of the buildings date from the 19th century. Brighton Place, a small square to the north of Market St, formerly called The Knab (Scandinavian for a hill, or a piece of rising ground), was the site of the town well and the venue for town meetings. Many of the cobble-fronted houses round the square have been demolished, but the old flint-fronted inn, the Druid's Head, a favourite resort of fishermen, still survives.

English's Oyster Bar (**28**), the celebrated fish restaurant at the entrance to the narrow alleyway of Market St, is one of the many Regency houses in Brighton to have had its ground floor altered to form shop windows, whilst retaining bays and other Regency features in its upper floor. In Edwardian times this was called the Cheeseman's Oyster Bar and was run by two imperious sisters. Smoking on the premises was strictly forbidden, as it might spoil the flavour of the oysters, and when Edward VII entered the restaurant one day smoking a cigar the sisters refused to serve him until he had put it out – which he did without protest.

The Bath Arms (**29**), at the corner of Meeting House Lane and Union St, one of the many popular drinking places in the Lanes, was built in the 1860s and has been restored to its original appearance, recreating its Victorian atmosphere.

▼28   29

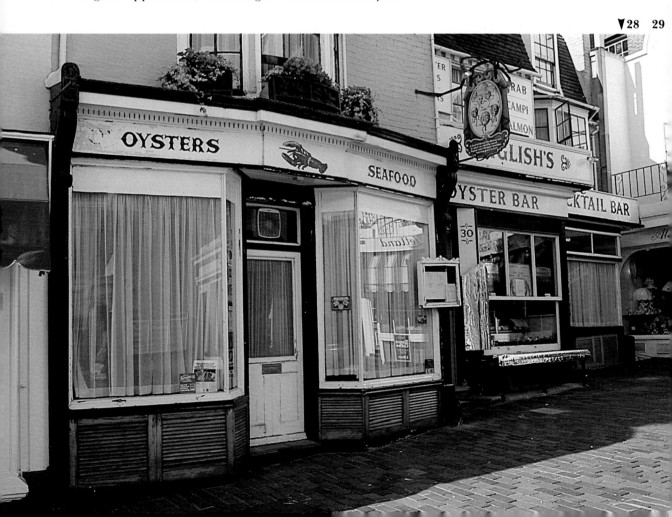

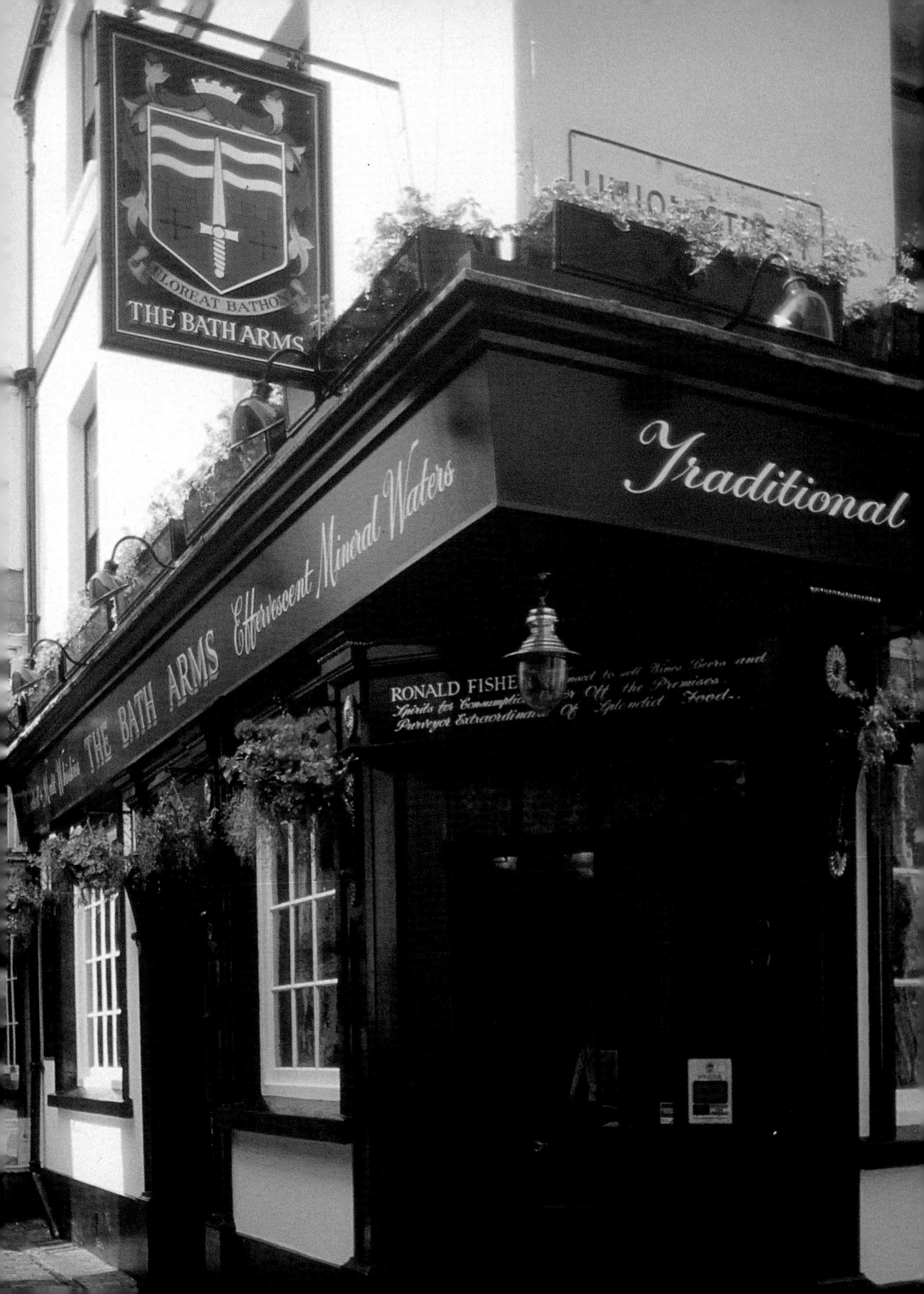

FLOREAT BATHON
THE BATH ARMS
THE BATH ARMS
Effervescent Mineral Waters
Traditional
RONALD FISHE

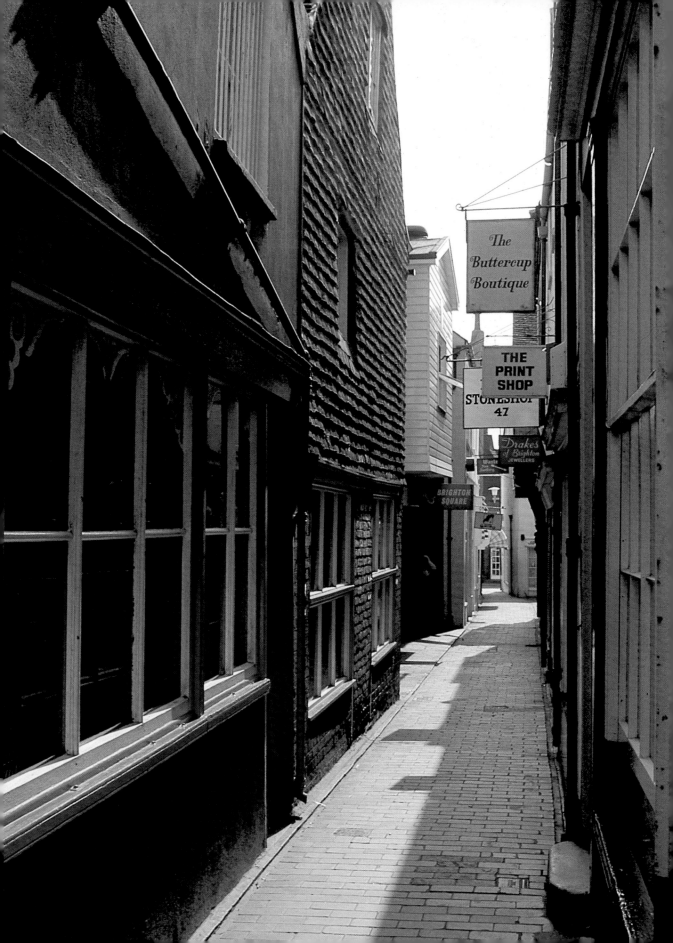

Meeting House Lane (**30**) takes its name from the Friends' Meeting House, which was built here in 1800 and altered and enlarged in 1876; there has been a community of Quakers in Brighton since the 17th century. At the corner of Meeting House Lane opposite the Bath Arms is the Elim Four Square Tabernacle, built by Amon Wilds in 1825 on the site of the earliest Nonconformist chapel in the town (1683).

The Cricketers' Arms (**31**) in Black Lion St is one of the most attractive of Brighton's old inns and has recently been refurbished. It was originally called The Last and Fish Cart, a last being equivalent to 10,000 fish; the doorway was inscribed 'Long time I've looked for good beer, And at "The Last" I've found it here'. In the 1790s, when it was a popular coaching inn, its name was changed by the landlord, Mr Jutton, a great cricket enthusiast. To the right of the pub is the inn yard – the last site of the town pound, and still used as such in the 1860s. To the left is the Derek Carver, a modern inn named after one of the first Protestant martyrs in the reign of Mary Tudor. Derek Carver came to England from Flanders to escape religious persecution; he became a prominent citizen and owner of the Black Lion Brewery (named after the Black Lion of Flanders), which stood on this site. In 1554 he was arrested after attending a prayer meeting in the town, and after several months in Newgate Prison he was burned at the stake at Lewes. He behaved with great courage at his execution, speaking to the assembled crowd and, when the fire was lit, throwing his Bible to the bystanders. His death is commemorated by a plaque on the wall of the new building.

0
1

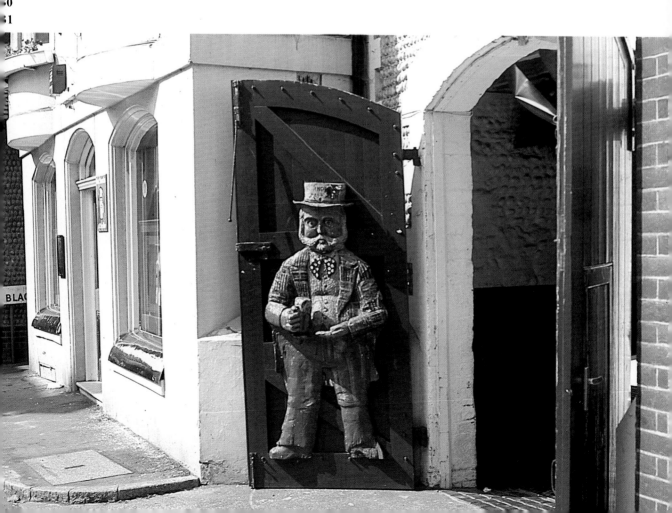

Ship St was built on the area known as the Hempshares (see p. 7), and became known as the Chancery Lane of Brighton because so many lawyers had their offices there. It takes its name from the Old Ship Hotel. This is the oldest inn in Brighton; the earliest reference to it dates from 1559, but its origins may go back further. With the Castle Hotel it became the social centre of the town in the 18th century, when Ship St was one of the main thoroughfares. Its Assembly Rooms, added to the back of the hotel building in 1775, were designed by Robert Golden in an Adamesque style. After the Castle closed balls and concerts continued to be held here, their popularity enhanced by the fact that Mrs Fitzherbert was their patroness for several years. The Assembly Rooms were also used for important town and business meetings, and for property sales. Today the hotel has been modernised and much enlarged, but it remains one of the most popular venues in the town. Ship St still has many of its 18th-century houses; particularly fine are nos. 61–62 (**34**), and no. 69 (**32**), one of the few houses in the centre of the town to be faced with knapped (split) flints, rather than the more traditional materials (see below).

The attractive little 37a, Duke St (**33**), lies hidden in a yard near the junction of Middle St and Duke St. Most unusually it is fronted with boarding; though this is common elsewhere in Sussex it is rare in Brighton, where cottages of this sort were generally faced with cobbles, the most readily available local material (in the case of Brighton these were pebbles picked up from the beach), tarred to protect them from harsh winds and sea spray. Windows and doorways were often surrounded by brick (painted cream to contrast with the black cobbling) to strengthen the structure; brick was used for a whole house only by the rich, as transport costs made it expensive – it had to be brought from the other side of the Downs.

▼ 32

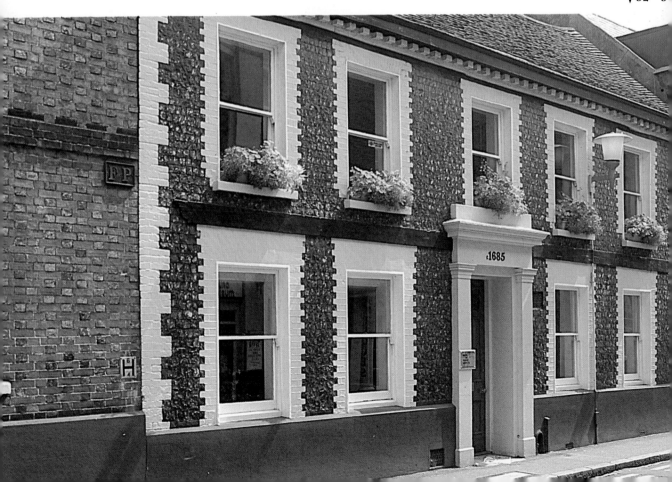

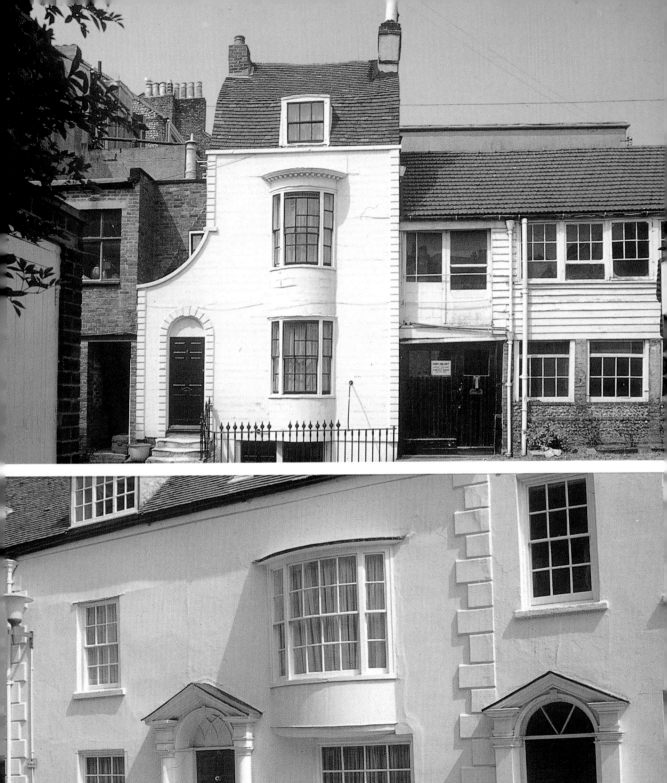
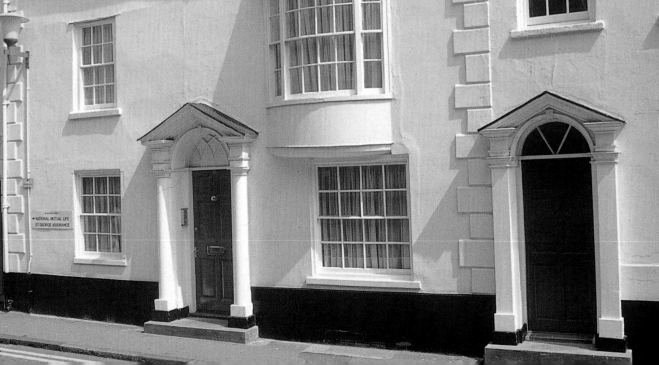

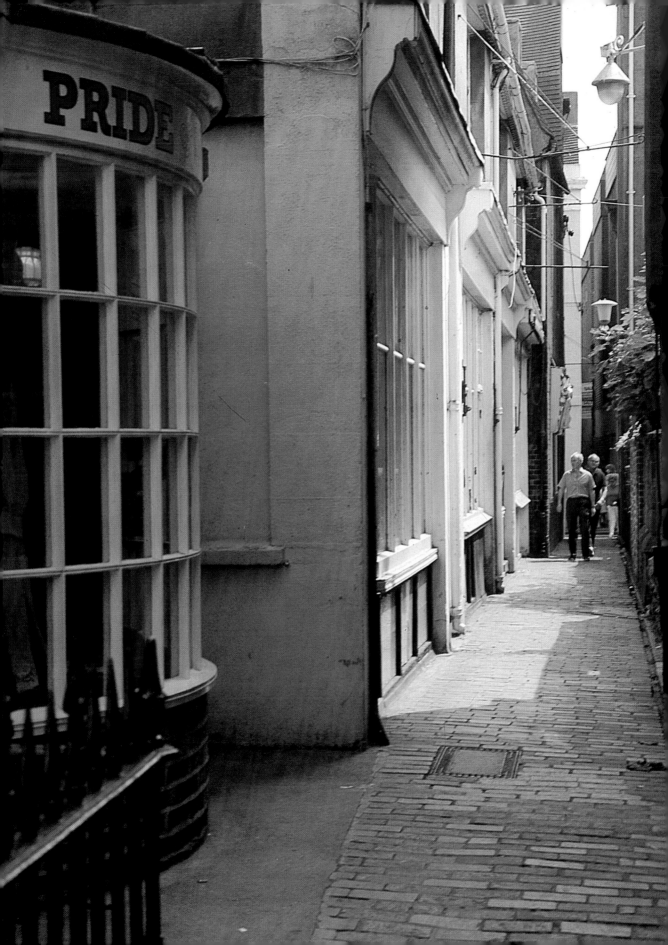

Ship St Gardens (**35**, **36**), the approach into the Lanes from the west, leads to Prince Albert St, the antique buyers' paradise. Brighton is one of the major centres of Britain's antique trade, and many shops in and around the Lanes sell goods of a variety paralleled in few places outside London; several of them, following the example of the Pavilion, specialise in spectacular pieces of Chinoiserie. Though it is not part of the Lanes proper, Ship St Gardens has the same colourful, intimate atmosphere. Its continuation, Black Lion Lane, is the site of some of the favourite local stories whose point is the narrowness of the Lanes. One of the best known concerns a very fat man who challenged a noted athlete to a race on condition that he could choose the course and be given a start of 10 yards: he chose Black Lion Lane and scored an easy victory, because there was no room for his opponent to overtake him. It is also related that the fugitive Charles II, at one point during his escape from Brighton, was carried down the Lane on the back of a fisherman. They encountered a stout fishwife, and, as he could not pass her and was afraid to go back, the fisherman knocked her down and then climbed over her, bearing his Royal burden to safety.

5

6

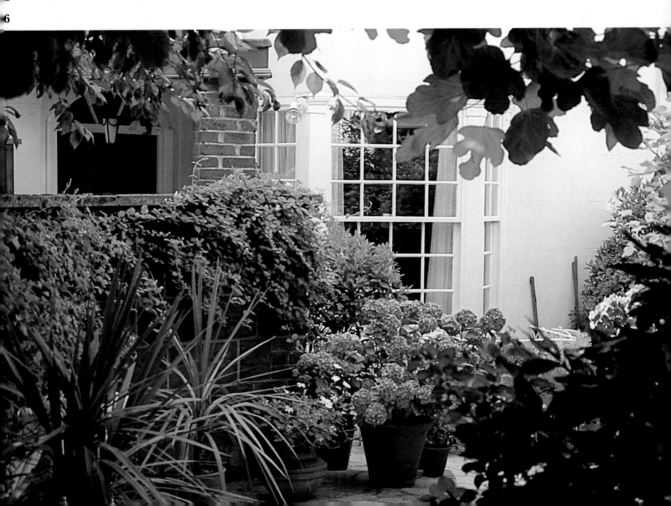

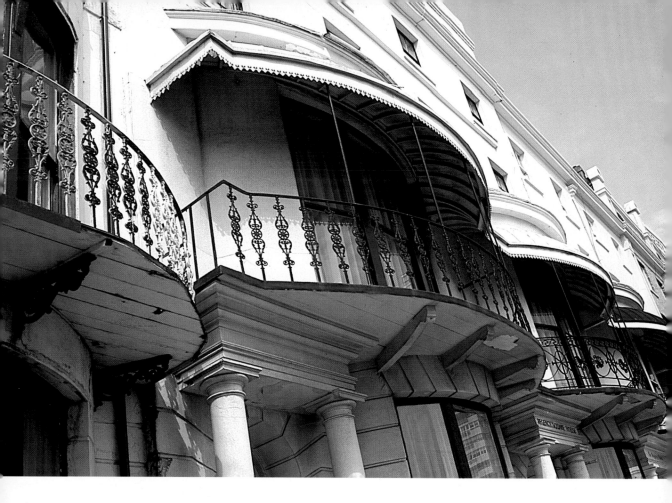

Regency Square (**37**) was laid out by Joshua Flesher Hanson in 1818 on land previously known as Belle Vue Fields, where fairs and military reviews were held. A windmill standing in the south-west corner of the field was moved in 1797 to a hill just outside Preston by 36 oxen (a print of this can be seen at Preston Manor), to raise the tone of the area for new residents. Many of the houses have the attractive hooded bow-fronted windows and elegant ironwork balconies characteristic of their period; the architect was probably Amon Wilds. St Albans House, in the south-west corner (now part of the Beach Hotel), was built after the others, having being designed by Amon Wilds' son, A. H. Wilds. Between 1830 and 1837 it was the home of the Duke and Duchess of St Albans; the Duchess had begun her career as the actress Harriet Mellon, and on the death of her first husband, the banker Thomas Coutts, she became the richest woman in England. The Duke of St Albans was 20 years her junior. She left her fortune to her granddaughter, Angela Burdett, who became Baroness Burdett-Coutts, the philanthropist.

Several of the early-19th-century Brighton squares were laid out to face inland; unfortunately the outlook of Russell Square (**38**) has been rather marred by the construction of a multi-storey car park right opposite. In itself however it is charming, with many of the architectural characteristics typical of the town but on a more modest scale than many of the squares. Some of the houses have been renovated, for example the one shown here: the bright blue of its balcony is unusual in Brighton, where the dominant colours are cream and pale yellow, and nicely evokes the gaiety of a seaside town.

7 38►

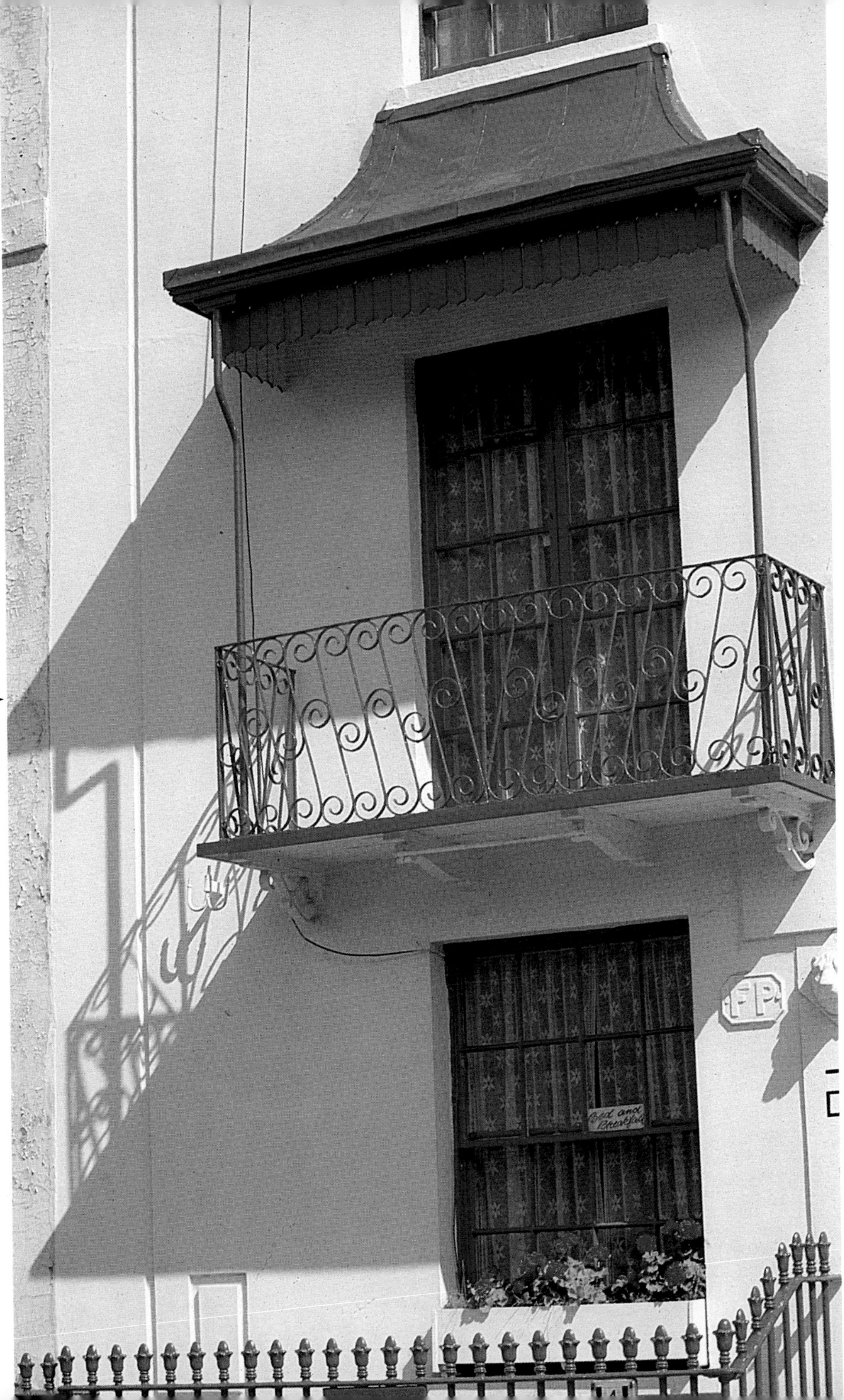

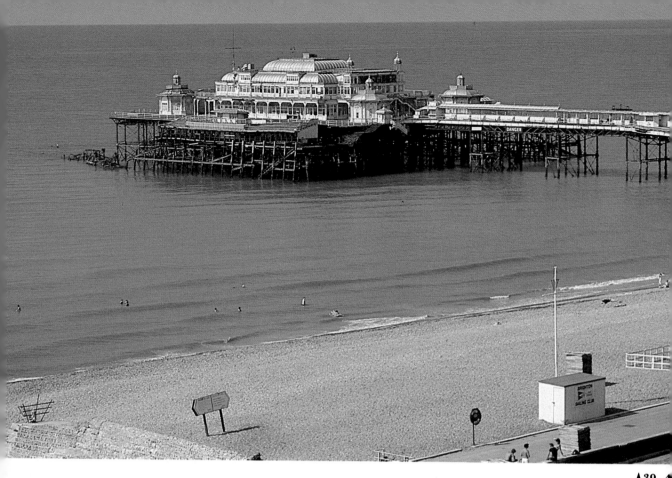

'As a means of recreation and health, nothing could be more advantageous, and the beautiful pier will remain as an example to future ages of what speculation has done in the 19th century', declared the Mayor of Brighton at the opening of the West Pier (**39**) in October 1866. The 19th century was the heyday of pier building: piers became fashionable places to promenade at the seaside. The West Pier, designed by Eusebius Birch, was one of the first to be opened – in defiance of opposition from the residents of Regency Square, who felt it would ruin their view of the sea. It was a great success, and attracted large numbers of visitors, besides providing a landing place for steamers. In the early 1890s it was nearly doubled in size by the addition of new landing stages and a concert hall. The pier was renowned for its sideshows which, in 1890, included a display of performing fleas, and a small cannon which was fired at noon every day by the effect of the sun's rays (when the sun shone). Many of the promenaders were visitors at the Grand (**40**) and other smart hotels in this part of the town, so the pier came to be regarded as more 'select' than the Palace Pier. Sadly, one can no longer stroll along the West Pier, as corrosion has made it unsafe and one section has been demolished. The West Pier Trust is actively fund-raising to restore this magnificent relic of the Victorian age. Under West Pier (**41**) are stalls and shops selling all manner of goods for tourists. Looking eastwards along King's Road, one can see the white stucco and ironwork balconies of the Grand Hotel and the concrete of the Brighton Centre. West of the Grand is the red brick and terracotta Metropole Hotel, built in 1888 to a design by Alfred Waterhouse, whose other work includes the Natural History Museum, London. At first it was considered a great eyesore, its harsh colour standing out from the white stucco and pale yellow brick of the other buildings. Some of its most attractive features, the characteristic Waterhouse French pavilion turrets and the little spire on the roof, have been masked by modern additions.

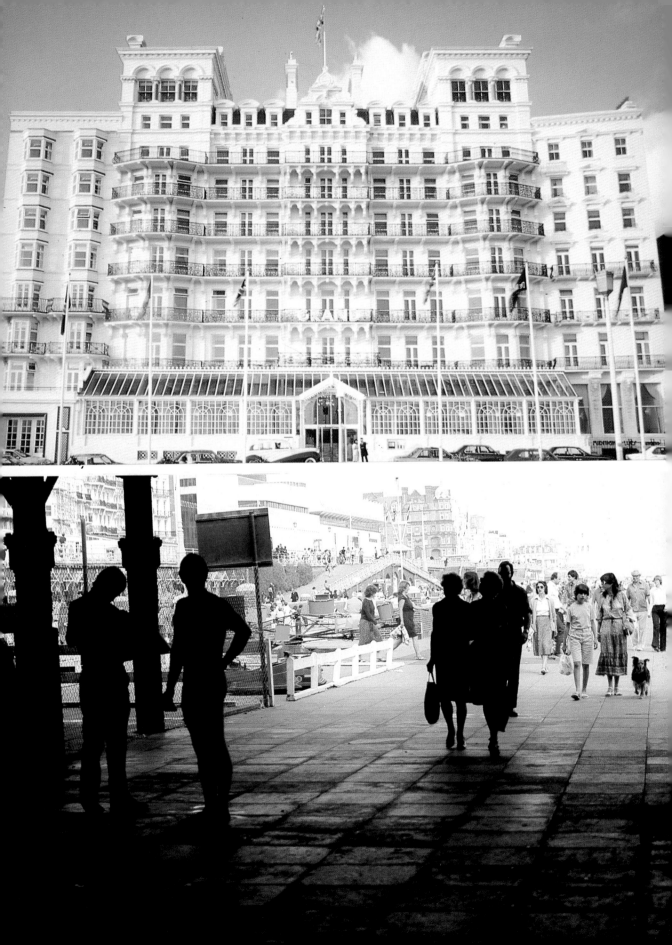

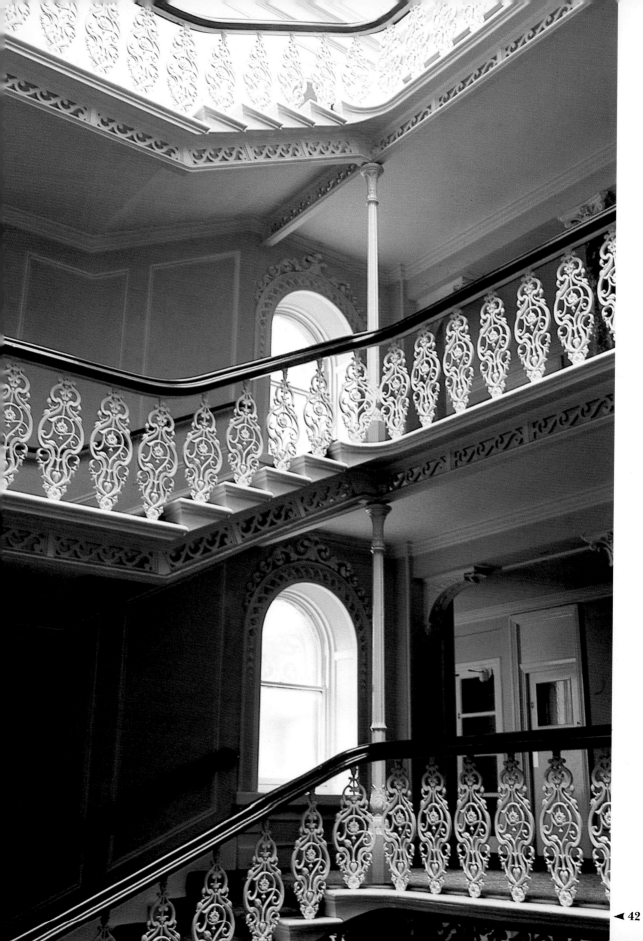

The Grand Hotel: **42**, the Staircase; **43**, the Dining Room, originally the Gentlemen's Coffee Room. By the mid-19th century fewer people wanted to rent a whole house for a stay in Brighton, and hotels were built to cater for their needs. The Grand, designed by J. H. Whichcord, was one of the first to be built and was also the most luxurious and the tallest: when it opened in 1864, the *Brighton Herald* declared that, with its nine stories towering above the other seafront buildings, 'it stands on our cliffs like Saul amidst the men of Israel'. According to the same newspaper report, republished by the hotel in 1977, constituents of the building included 3,500,000 bricks, 450 tons of wrought and cast iron, 1½ acres of glazed tiles, 15 miles of wallpaper, 230 marble chimney pieces, and 12 miles of bell wire; there were 260 rooms and the cost was £160,000. There were many 'Italian' features, including Florentine arches over windows and doorways. This was one of the first hotels in England to be fitted with electric light and lifts, or 'ascending omnibuses', as they were called, for guests. In the 1960s the Grand had fallen into disrepair and was threatened with demolition, but the government refused to countenance such an action and the hotel was restored, both inside and out, to its Victorian splendour. It was beautifully restored again from the destruction caused by a bomb intended to eliminate the Conservative cabinet in 1984. Other fashionable hotels in the late 19th century included the Norfolk, the Bedford (Dickens' favourite) and the Royal Albion. For the less affluent there sprang up a large number of guest houses and lodging houses, ruled over by that indomitable British institution, the landlady.

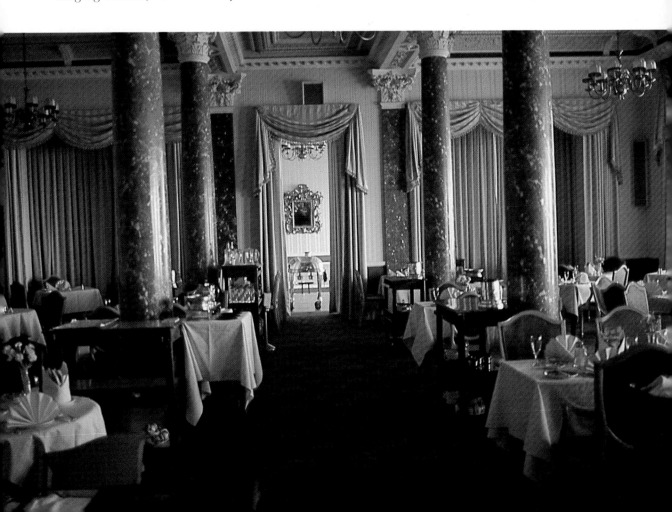

# Around the Centre from West to East

Building started at Brunswick Square (**45**), in the then tiny village of Hove, in 1824, inspired by the development of Kemp Town (see **53**). The designs were provided by Amon Wilds and C. A. Busby (see p. 17), the leading role being taken by Busby. Together with Brunswick Terrace this estate, Brunswick Town, was intended to be self-supporting; small houses for tradespeople were built adjoining the square, and a church and a closed market were also erected. By the Brunswick Square Act (1830), commissioners were appointed to regulate the estate's affairs; these later became the Hove Commissioners and subsequently Hove Corporation. The part of the Act stipulating that all the houses of the estate be repainted in a uniform colour every three years is still in force. Visitors who stayed in Brunswick Town included Prince Metternich, the exiled Austrian chancellor, who, like several European statesmen and royal personages, took up residence in Brighton after the wave of revolutions that swept through Europe in 1848. Adelaide Crescent (**44**), named after William IV's queen, was begun in 1830; the architect was Decimus Burton. Only 10 houses were constructed at first, the rest of the crescent being left incomplete for 50 years. The difference in design can be clearly seen, the houses added later (those on the eastern side) having much plainer facades and far less charm.

OVERLEAF: the King and Queen Inn (**46**), Marlborough Place, acquired its 'Tudor' appearance in the 1930s, when all its Regency features were destroyed. Before the 1780s it was a farmhouse outside the town proper, and until 1868 it served as the Cornmarket. Formerly barracks backed on to the inn, and drink used to be smuggled to the soldiers through a hole in the wall. The King and Queen, now Henry VIII and Anne Boleyn to fit the Tudor image, were probably originally George III and Queen Charlotte. **47**: one end of Montpelier Crescent. The main sweep of the crescent shows A. H. Wilds' work on its grandest scale. Some of the mansions have his characteristic pilasters with 'Ammonite' capitals, so called because of the resemblance of their volutes to fossil ammonites.

▼**44** 4:

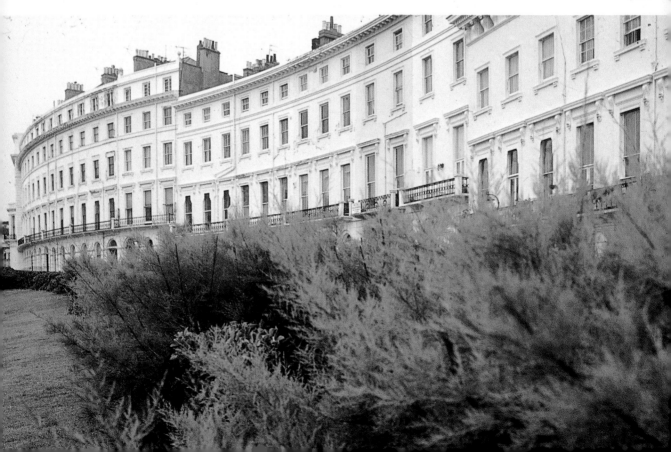

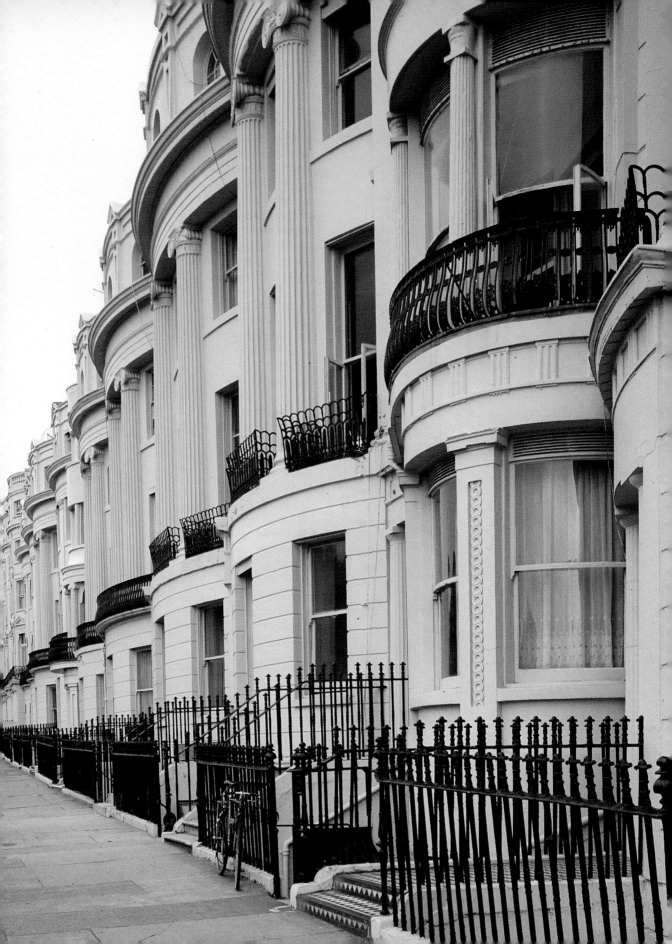

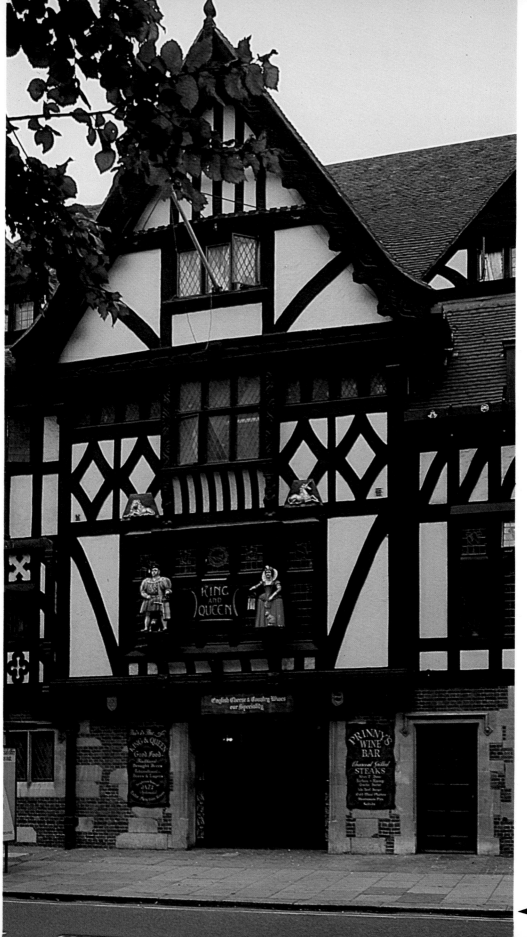

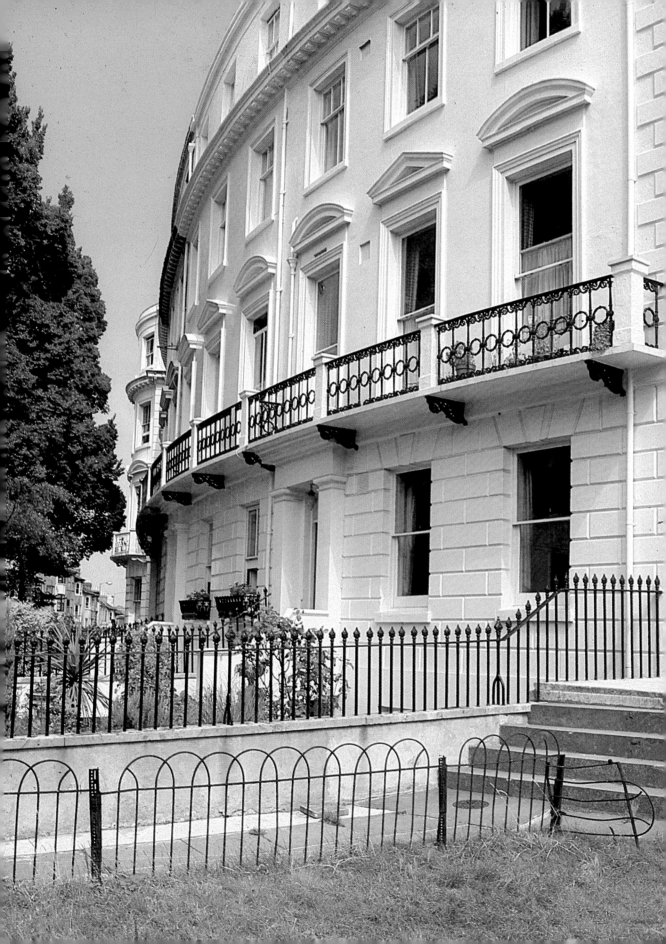

The lively Saturday market in Upper Gardener St (**48**, **49**) sells all manner of bric-a-brac and second-hand clothes as well as fresh vegetables and fruit, and always attracts flocks of Brighton visitors and residents. This area grew up in the early 19th century. As elsewhere in Brighton, the alignment of the streets was largely determined by the Brighton tenantry laines – arable fields on the edge of the town which were generally subdivided into furlongs separated by narrow pathways known as leakways. When the land came to be built on, speculators tended to develop it a furlong at a time; long rows of houses covered the strips of fields and the leakways became the main streets. The houses were occupied mainly by artisans, who came here in growing numbers after the railway opened. The area was ill-drained and overcrowded, but since the 1970s it has become fashionable. The more derelict terraces have been demolished, and many of the remaining ones have been 'done up'. The cottage character of the houses makes them popular with young families, in preference to the vast Regency houses on the seafront, many of which are now converted into flats for old people and students or used as hotels.

▼48  4

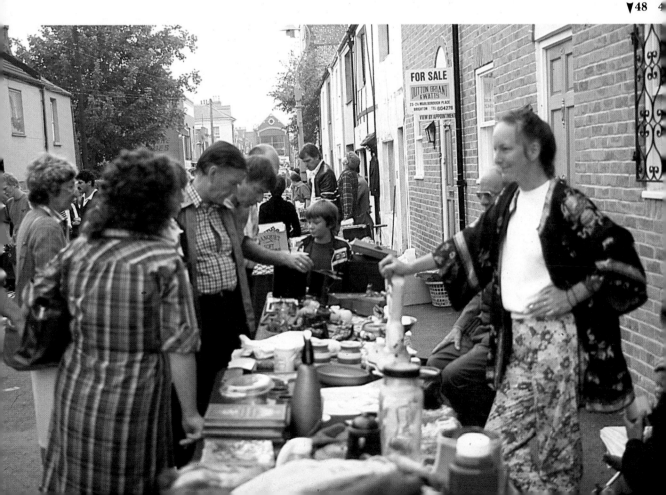

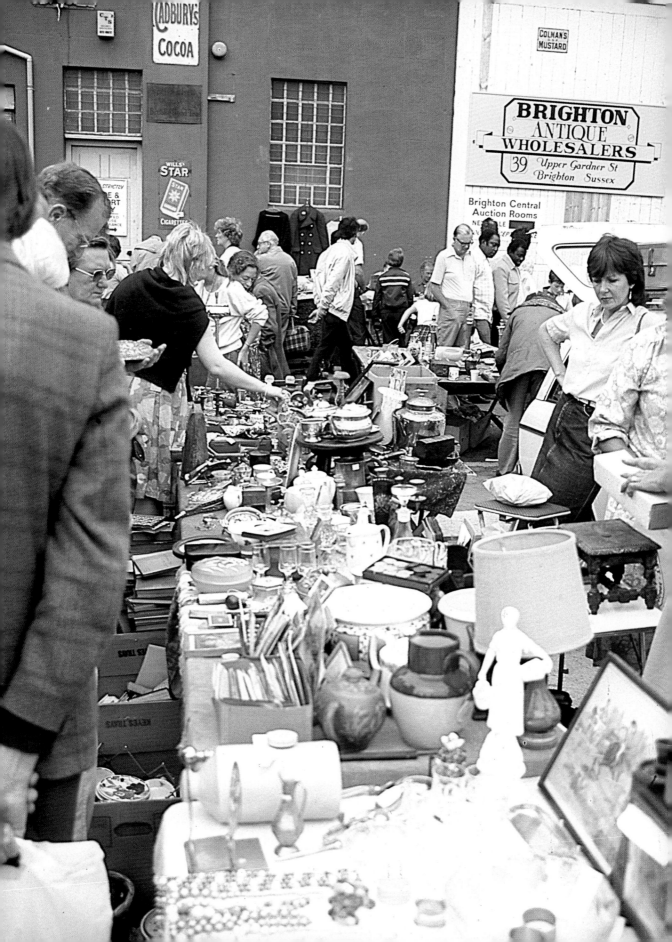

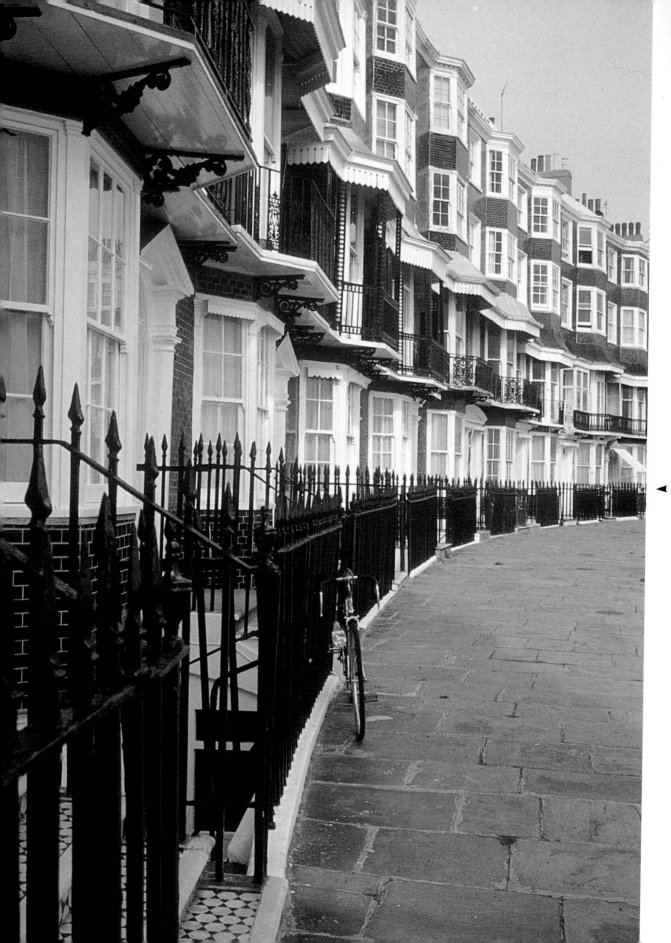

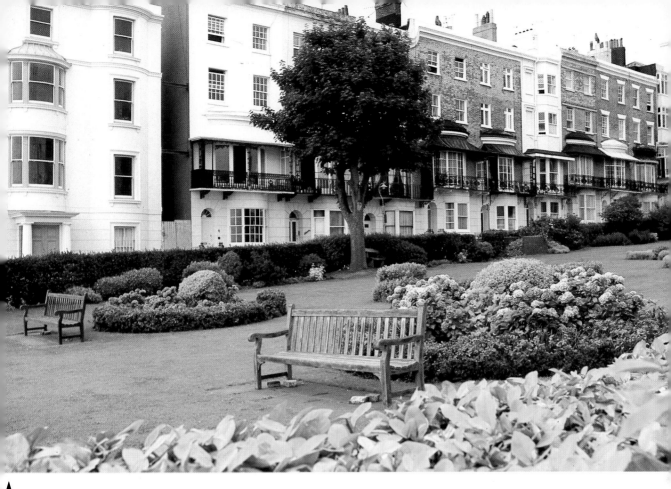

The Royal Crescent (**50**), completed in 1807, was the first of the many early-19th-century housing schemes in Brighton to be planned as a single architectural whole. The building was financed by J. B. Otto, a West Indian speculator; the architect is unknown. The houses form a distinctive and delightful group, standing on the cliff top facing the sea, all fronted with 'mathematical' tiles (see also **19**). They all have four stories, ironwork balconies with bonnet-like canopies and doorways with broken pediments, yet they vary considerably in size and internal structure. When the crescent was finished and its name was being added above the centre houses the workman performing the task leaned back, presumably to examine his work, overbalanced, and fell to his death on the railings below. At one time a statue of the Prince Regent by the sculptor Rossi stood in the middle of the grass enclosure in front of the crescent; Otto erected it to gain favour with the Prince. However it did not have the desired effect, being much disliked by the Regent, and as it was of inferior stone it soon began to crumble, one of the arms disintegrating first, which made people think that it was of Lord Nelson; eventually it was removed (1819).

Much seaside architecture has been influenced by the attraction of the sea itself – people have wanted to be able to see the sea, hence the three-sided squares, the bow windows and the balconies of Brighton. Marine Square (**51**) was built about 1824, inspired, as was so much of the building in this period, by the development of Kemp Town to the east. It was laid out by Thomas Attree, a well-known local figure from a family firm of solicitors whose clients included the Prince Regent (the firm acted for him in the purchases of land for the Pavilion estate). The houses are rather a jumble of details, with a great variety of balconies and verandas, and all with attractive bow windows on the ground and first floors. The eastern side of the terrace has been largely spoiled by modernisation.

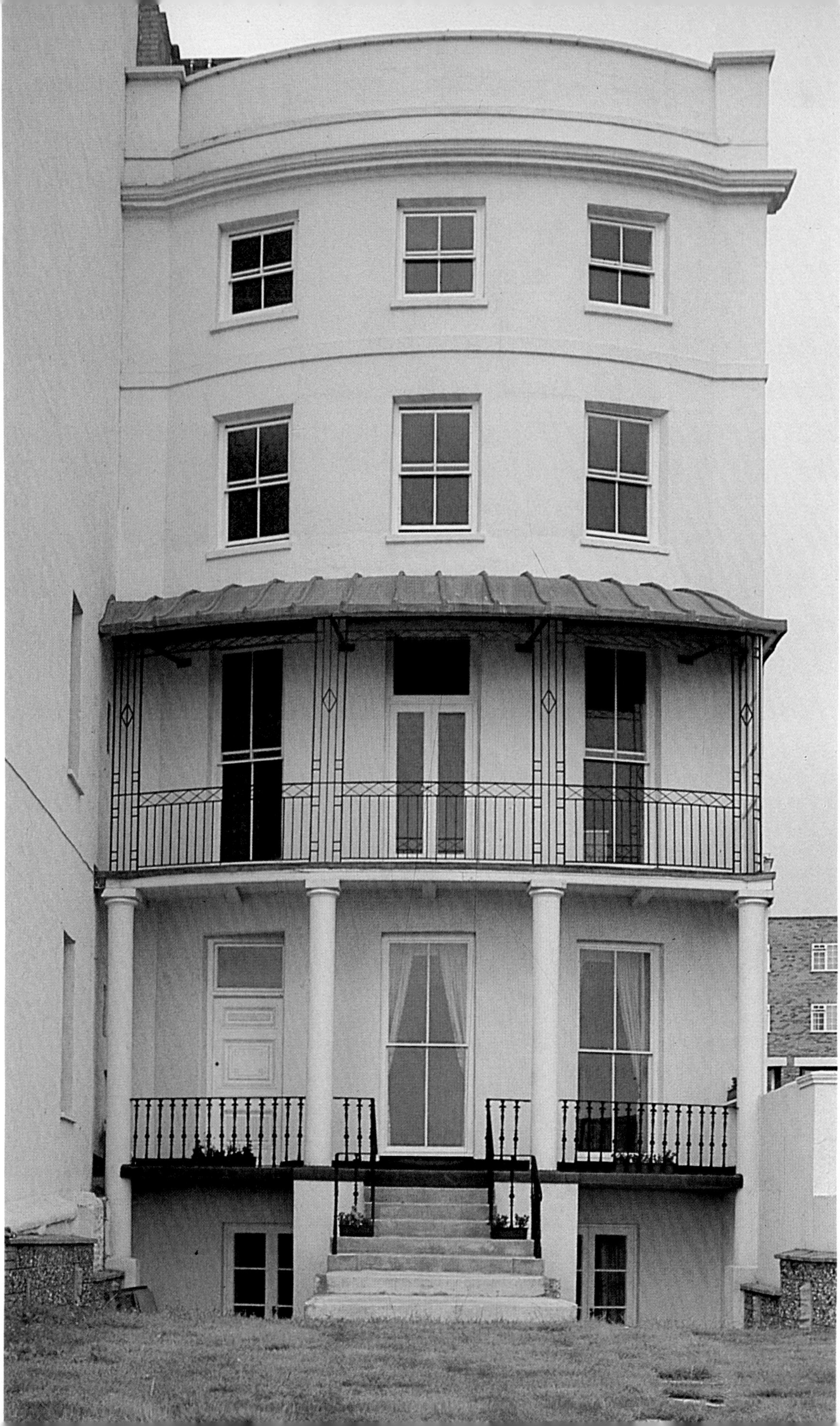

◄52 5

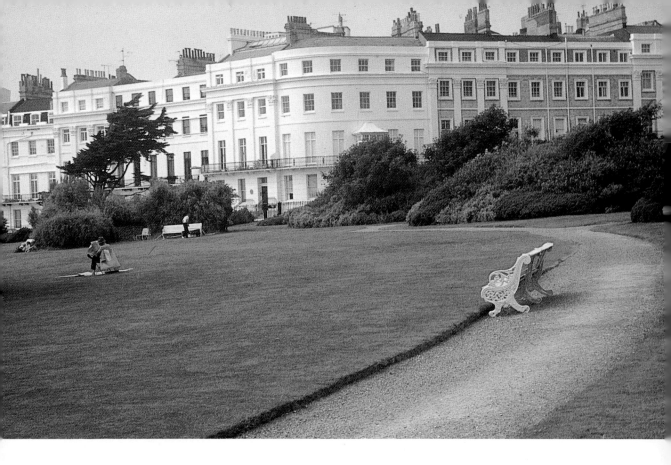

Originally the Brighton–Rottingdean road ran along the seafront east of Old Steine, with a stretch of rough fenced ground to the south of it on the cliff edge. When the town spread eastwards this stretch was called East Cliff and, later, Marine Parade. Houses were built along it from about 1800, and despite Victorian and later alteration and rebuilding, many retain their original character. No. 140 (**52**) is one of the most elegant; its attractive balcony is supported on Doric columns, with a railing of plain uprights topped by St Andrew crosses. Like many of the houses on the Parade it was designed by Wilds and Busby.

Lewes Crescent (**53**) is the centre of the grand architectural scheme of Kemp Town, devised by Thomas Read Kemp, a wealthy local landowner and sometime MP for nearby Lewes; he was inspired by Nash's Regent's Park, London, to create a similar development for wealthy residents and visitors in Brighton. Building started in 1823. The main part of the estate consists of Sussex Square, the huge Lewes Crescent (its span is enormous, 840 ft – 200 ft wider than the Royal Crescent in Bath) and, on either side of it, Chichester and Arundel Terraces. Kemp originally intended the estate to be twice its present size, but his money ran out. The architects, Wilds and Busby, were responsible only for the general layout and for the façades; the interiors and backs of the houses were left to be completed by the proprietors, so no two are exactly the same. But the scheme did not take at first, and by 1834 only 34 of the 105 houses were occupied. Kemp went bankrupt and fled the country, just before he was declared an outlaw in Brighton. Later the estate became fashionable. In the mid-19th century, at 1, Lewes Crescent, and the adjacent 14, Chichester Terrace, the Duke of Devonshire entertained Palmerston, Thackeray and Landseer, and Edward VII stayed here with his daughter the Duchess of Fife in 1908. The garden enclosure in front of Lewes Crescent was laid out by the local botanist Henry Philips; the shrubs have been swept into strange shapes by the strong sea wind.

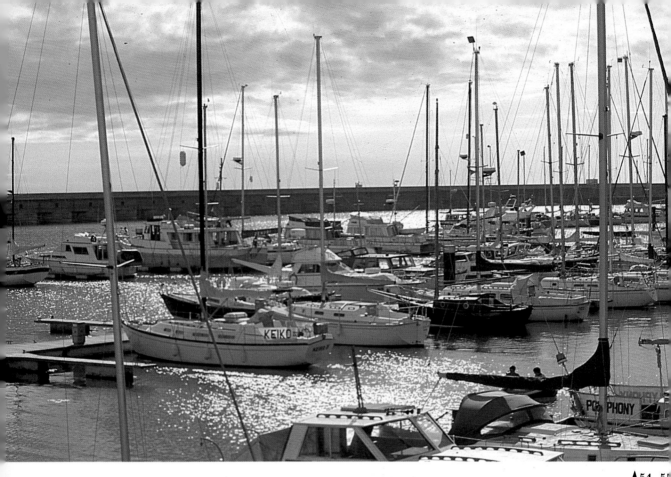

Modern developments in Brighton: **54** and **55**, the Marina; **56**, the Brighton Centre. The idea of building a marina in Brighton was first mooted in the 19th century, but it was not until the boom years of the 1960s that plans began to be implemented. The inspiration for the Marina at Black Rock came from Mr Harry Cohen, a local garage owner and keen yachtsman. The original plans were extremely ambitious and included provision for a heliport, a casino, a block of luxury flats and a conference hall, but the escalating costs of the venture (estimated to have risen 1200% in a decade) and vigorous objection by local preservation societies scotched most of these schemes. In fact the Marina has proved to be a very emotive issue, in Brighton and nationally: there were two town polls, two planning enquiries and debates on private members' bills in both Houses of Parliament before the project was allowed to go ahead. When eventually the Queen opened the Marina in May 1979 only the harbour facilities were complete. The massive harbour walls, encircling 77 acres of sheltered water, made it the largest marina in Europe. It is a thriving concern and has proved popular not only with sailors but also with fishermen (**55**). The development was finally completed with the provision of shops and restaurants in 1990.

Designed by the architects Russell Diplock Associates and built at a cost of over £9,000,000, the Brighton Centre occupies a prime position, on the seafront. It was opened in 1977 as part of Brighton's drive to establish itself as the premier conference venue in Britain. (Conferences are also held at the Dome – where one of the first ever annual conferences, that of the British Association for the Advancement of Science, was held in 1874 – and at the Hotel Metropole's Exhibition Centre.) The Centre provides excellent and highly versatile facilities: the huge main hall seats up to 5,120; the smaller Hewison Hall holds 800; the new East Wing holds 600 in each of its two rooms; and there are advanced communication facilities, with 4 camera rooms for the media and 8 interpreting rooms for simultaneous translation.

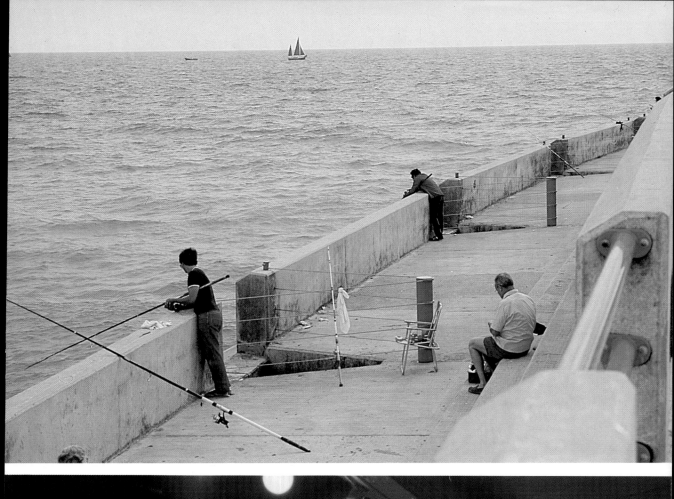

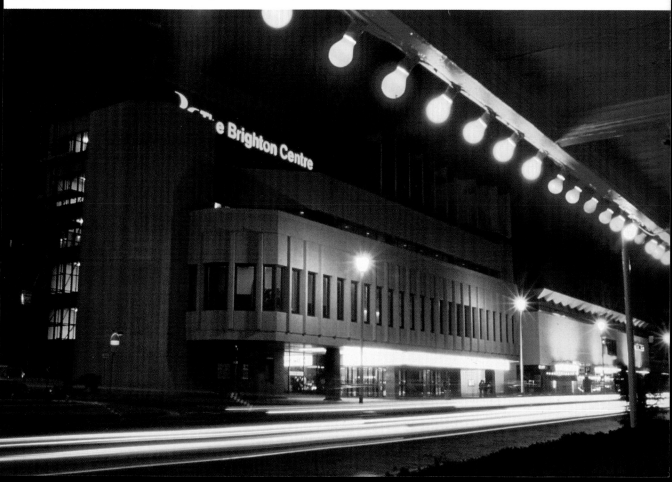

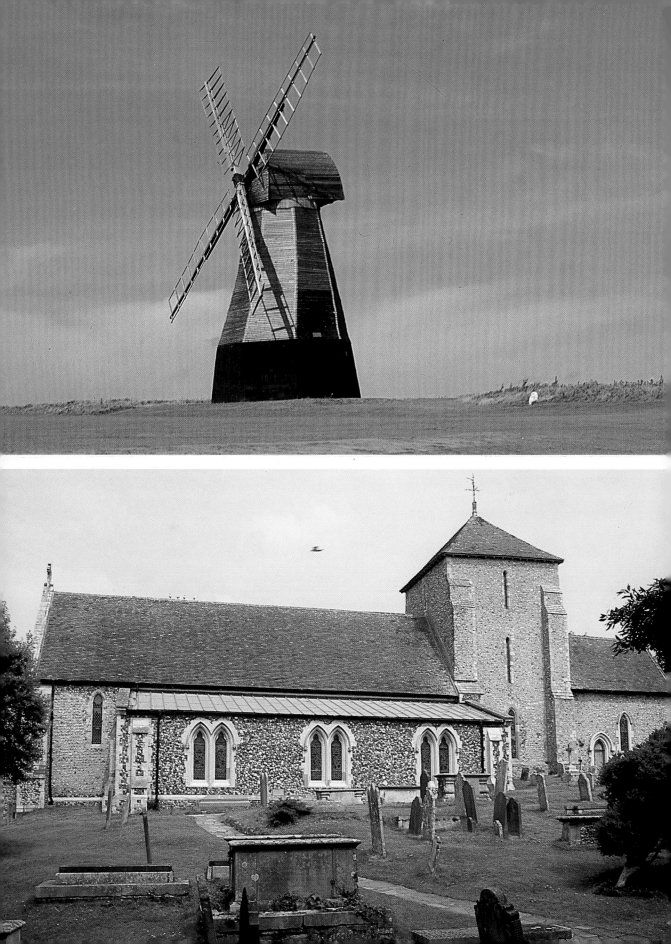

# The Villages from East to West

The small coastal farming community of Rottingdean became a fashionable adjunct to Brighton in the early 20th century, and there was much building along the shore. The village nevertheless retains its peaceful charm in the area around the green, at the north end of the High St. East of the green is St Margaret's church (**58**), mainly 13th century. In 1377 a French raiding party plundered and fired the village, and many villagers were burned alive in the belfry where they had taken refuge. The heat fractured flints in the church walls, and may be the reason for the odd pink and grey colouring of the arches and windows. In this century a group of Americans wanted to buy St Margaret's and take it back to the USA stone by stone; their attempt failed but they built an exact replica in their native Glendale, California, and named it The Church of the Recessional, after the poem by Rudyard Kipling, who lived in Rottingdean, at The Elms, between 1897 and 1903. Timbers (**59**), an excellent example of the conversion of an old Sussex barn into a dwelling, was formerly the main barn of West Side Farm, of which Hillside (**7**) was the farmhouse. Rottingdean Windmill (**57**), a fine 18th-century smock mill, is a prominent landmark on Beacon Hill, west of the village.

OVERLEAF: St Margaret's: the interior. The altar window (**60**), made by Morris & Co, was designed and given by Edward Burne-Jones in 1893 to mark his daughter Margaret's wedding in the church. It depicts the archangels Gabriel, Michael and Raphael, and, below, the Annunciation, Michael slaying the dragon, and the Guardian of little children. Four other windows in the church were also made by the Morris factory to Burne-Jones' designs. The particularly beautiful lancet window in the south side of the tower (**61**) represents the Tree of Jesse and shows Jesse, David, Solomon, Hezekiah, Jonah, and the Virgin and Child. Burne-Jones lived in Rottingdean at North End House from 1880 until his death in 1898; his ashes are buried in the churchyard.

7
8
9

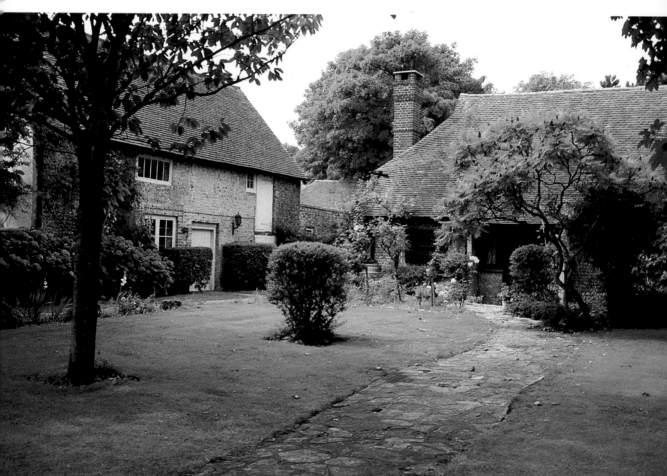

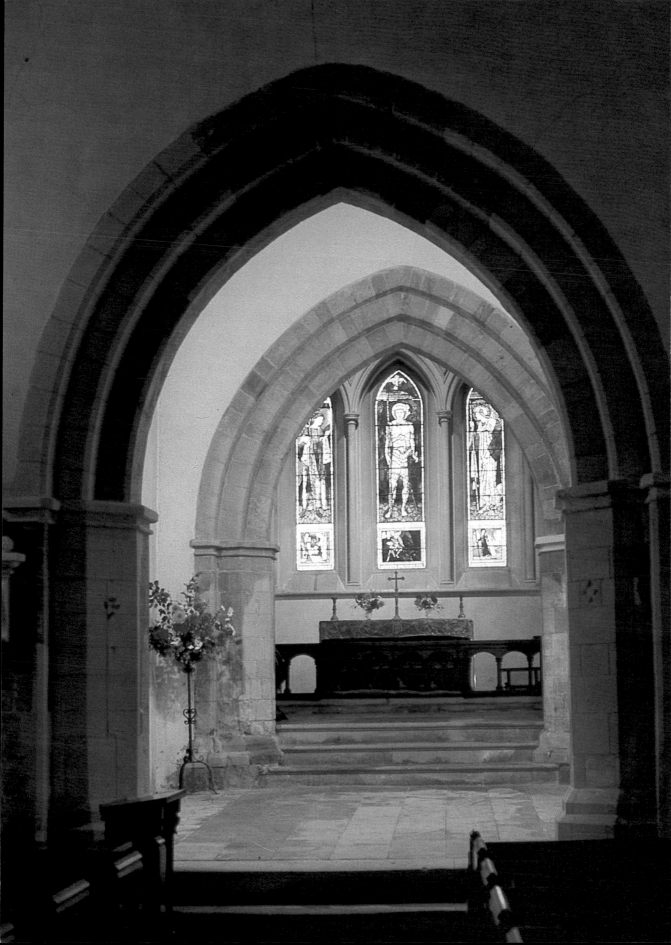

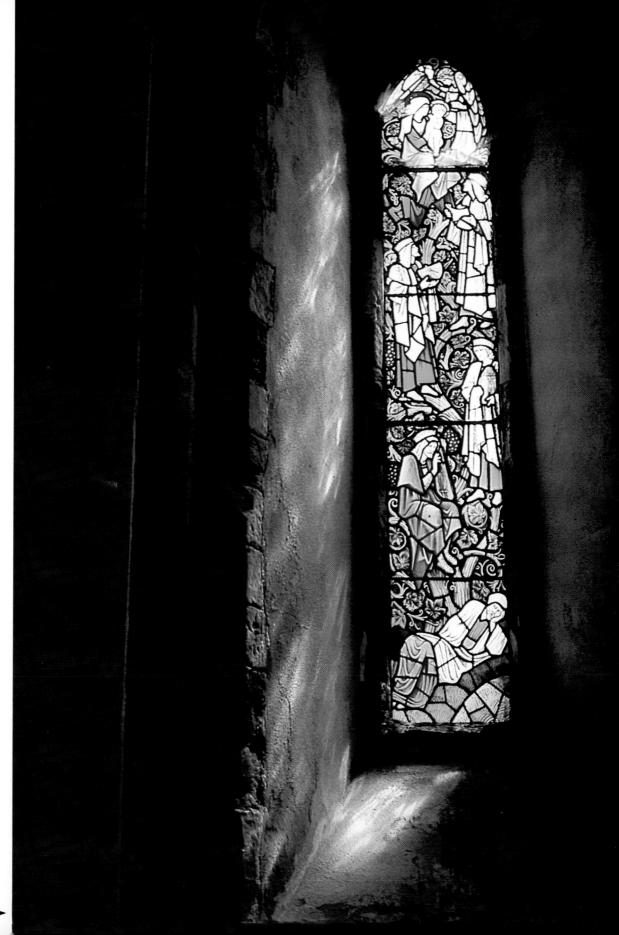

Though Preston village has been obliterated by the spread of Brighton, its identity survives in St Peter's church and Preston Manor. The layout of the delightful gardens of Preston Manor (**62**) is essentially Victorian and Edwardian, but there are some earlier features, such as the sunken garden surrounded by a ha-ha (probably late 18th century) and the walls round the walled garden, which date in part from 1250. Preston Manor House, on the site of a medieval manor, is a mainly 18th-century building, with early-20th-century additions. It now belongs to Brighton Corporation and houses the Thomas-Stanford Museum (named after the Manor's previous owner), a splendid collection of furniture, silver, china and paintings set out so as to give an impression of the house as it was in Edwardian times. The Corporation bought Preston Park in the 1880s for £50,000 to save it from property developers, and today these grounds are full of well-tended flowerbeds and provide such amenities as tennis courts, recreation grounds and playing fields for local residents.

The 13th-century parish church of St Peter (**62**, **63**) is so near to the Manor because in the 16th century the tenant was allowed to add part of the churchyard to his orchard in return for repairing the churchyard walls. Like many Sussex churches, it is of flint with stone dressing. Its chief glory, a wealth of 13th-century wall painting, suffered badly in a fire in 1906, and now only fragments remain: a Nativity scene on the north wall, and the murder of Thomas à Becket on one side of the chancel arch and a detail of the weighing of souls at the Last Judgement on the other. The paintings were whitewashed over in the 16th century and not rediscovered until the 18th.

▼62  6

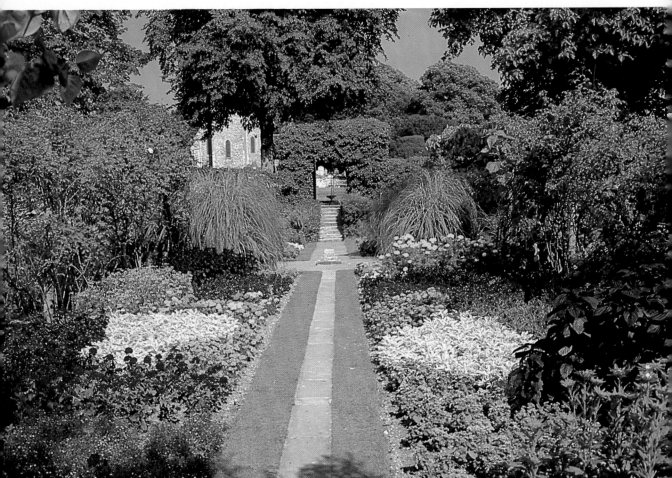

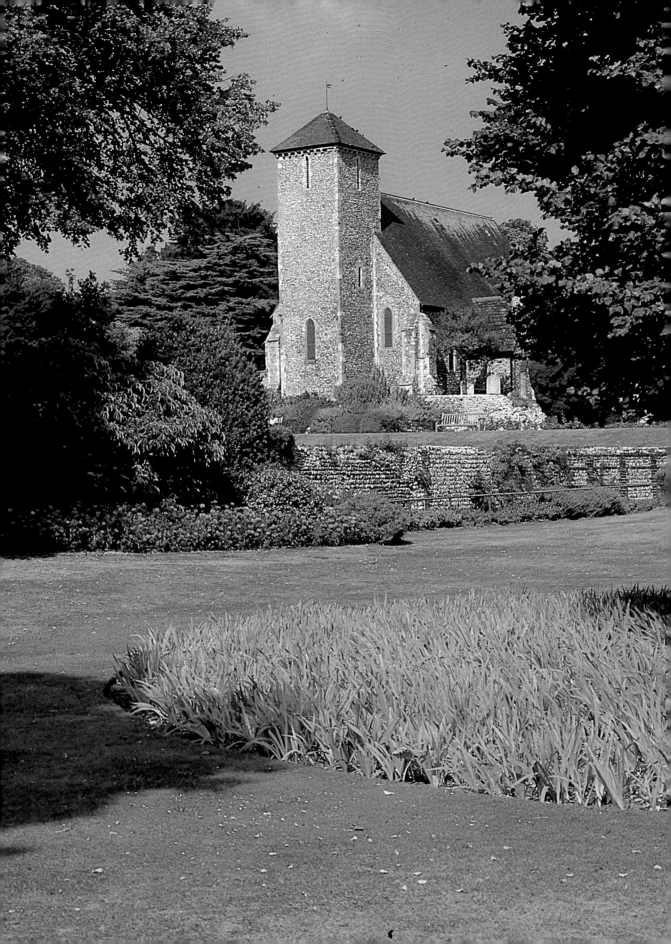

Only a few yards from the busy London–Brighton road lies the village of Patcham. Though now largely swallowed up by Brighton it still retains its own charm, especially in the centre of the village. In the Domesday Book (1086), Patcham is mentioned as Piceham, a manor belonging to William de Warenne; in those days it was a larger and more important settlement than the tiny village of Brighthelmeston which became Brighton. The main part of the village is now contained in the area around the steep Church Hill, on which stands a delightful row of cottages (**66**), some of them dating from the 15th century. They are built of a variety of local materials including brick and flint, with both tiled and slate roofs. In the early 1960s these cottages were threatened with demolition but, thanks to the action of the Patcham Preservation Society and Brighton Corporation, they were spared and skillfully restored, and are now under a preservation order. The church still has its Norman interior, with a (restored) 13th-century depiction of the Last Judgement above the chancel arch.

Patcham Place (**64**), the 'big house' of the village, is Elizabethan in origin but now presents a splendid 18th-century exterior, being faced (unusually for so large a dwelling) with black 'mathematical' tiles, which contrast strikingly with the white of the quoins, the window frames, the cornice and the doorway. In the 17th century the house was owned by the Stapley family, and was the home of Anthony Stapley, one of the signatories of Charles I's death warrant. Now it is a Youth Hostel, and has proved popular with walkers of the South Downs Way.

Southdown House (**65**), an attractive early Georgian house of knapped flint and brick, stands near the end of the London Road.

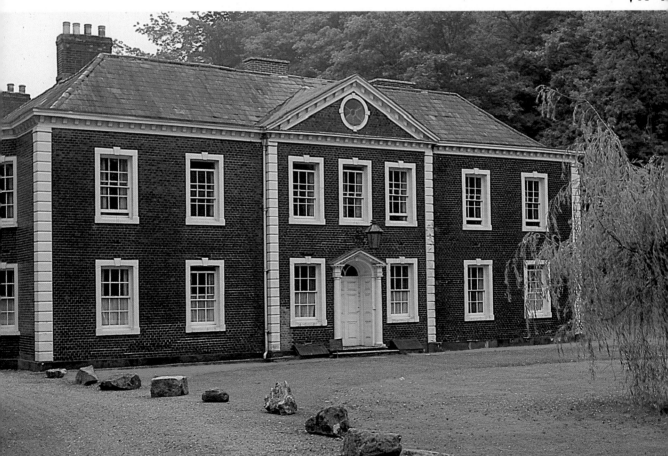

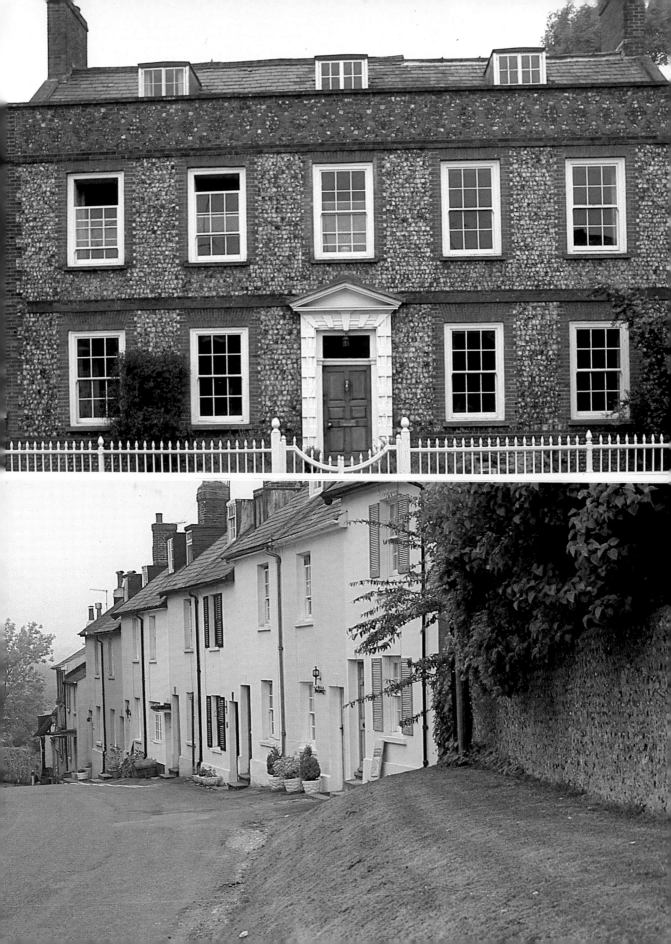

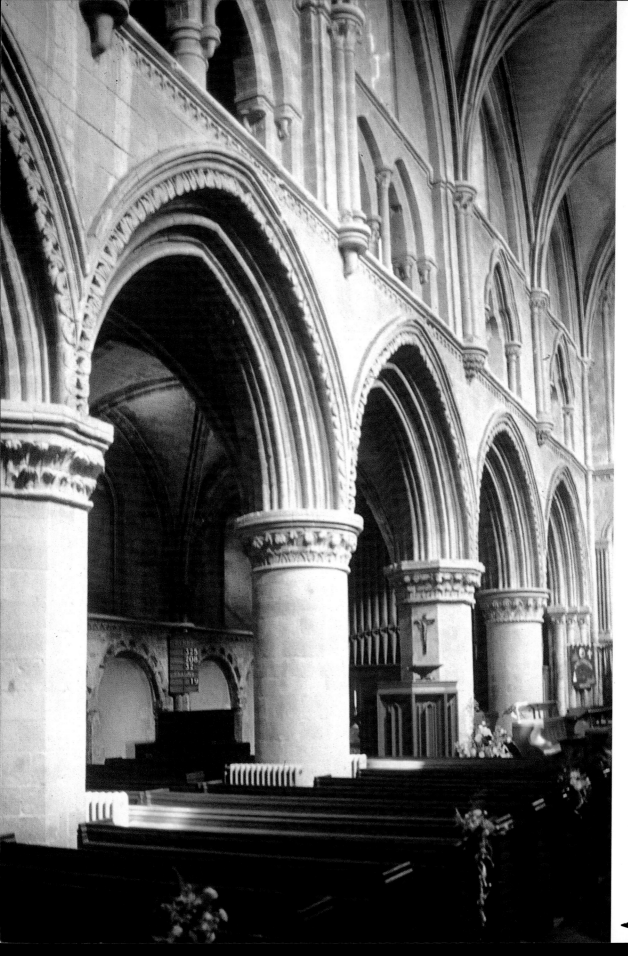

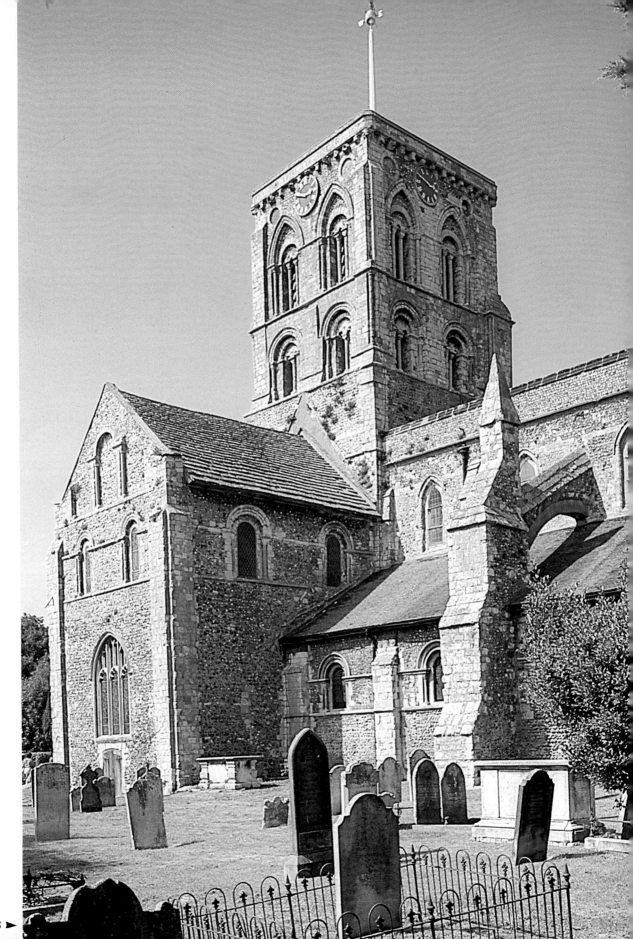

PRECEDING PAGES: The town and harbour of New Shoreham, known since 1910 as Shoreham by Sea, were laid out by the Normans about 1100. During the 12th and 13th centuries Shoreham was one of the chief ports of the south coast, and it is still the main port of Sussex. Dominating the town is the striking building of the church of St Mary de Haura (i.e. de Havre, of the harbour), probably the finest medieval church in Sussex (**67**, **68**). It was built between 1100 and 1225, in a mixture of Norman and transitional styles, which admirably demonstrate how the Norman style evolved into Gothic. Originally the church was twice its present length, enormous for a parish church, but the nave lay in ruins by the 17th century – why is uncertain: the damage may have been done during the struggles of the Civil War, or perhaps it was inflicted by a French raiding party in 1628. The tower, 81 ft high, soars above other buildings in the sprawling town, while the weight of the church is supported by magnificent Early English flying buttresses. The congregation is now confined to what was originally the choir. The two magnificent arcades, each of five bays, are of different formations although probably contemporary. The north arcade, shown here, has pillars of alternately round and octagonal columns, their capitals carved with stiff-leaf foliage. The south arcade has compound pillars with column shafts (probably of a slightly later date than the pillars) reaching in an unbroken line to the fine vaulting of the roof.

Empty deck chairs at the end of the day, with the lengthening shadows of the evening sun echoing the stripes on their canvas.

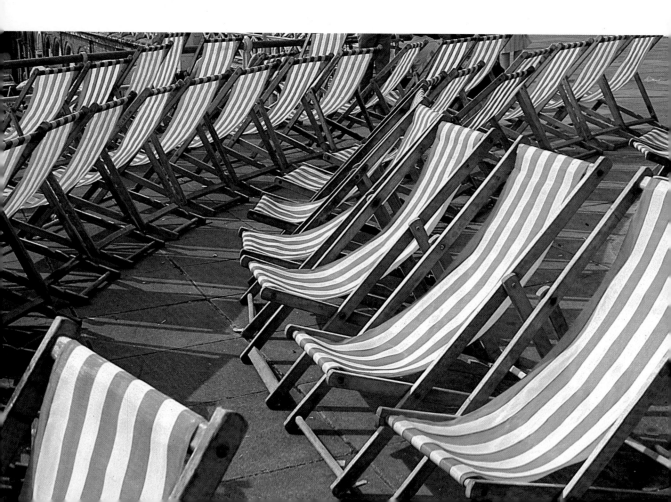

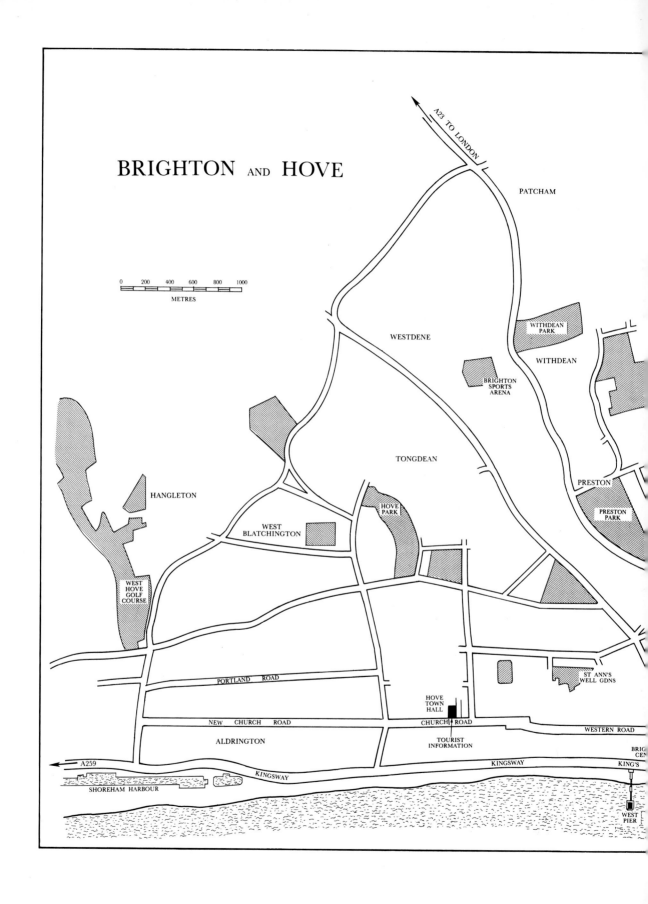

# BRIGHTON AND HOVE

0  200  400  600  800  1000
METRES

A23 TO LONDON

PATCHAM

WITHDEAN PARK

WITHDEAN

WESTDENE

BRIGHTON SPORTS ARENA

TONGDEAN

PRESTON

PRESTON PARK

HANGLETON

HOVE PARK

WEST BLATCHINGTON

WEST HOVE GOLF COURSE

ST ANN'S WELL GDNS

PORTLAND ROAD

HOVE TOWN HALL

CHURCH ROAD

WESTERN ROAD

NEW CHURCH ROAD

ALDRINGTON

TOURIST INFORMATION

A259

KINGSWAY

KINGSWAY

BRIG CEN

KING'S

SHOREHAM HARBOUR

WEST PIER

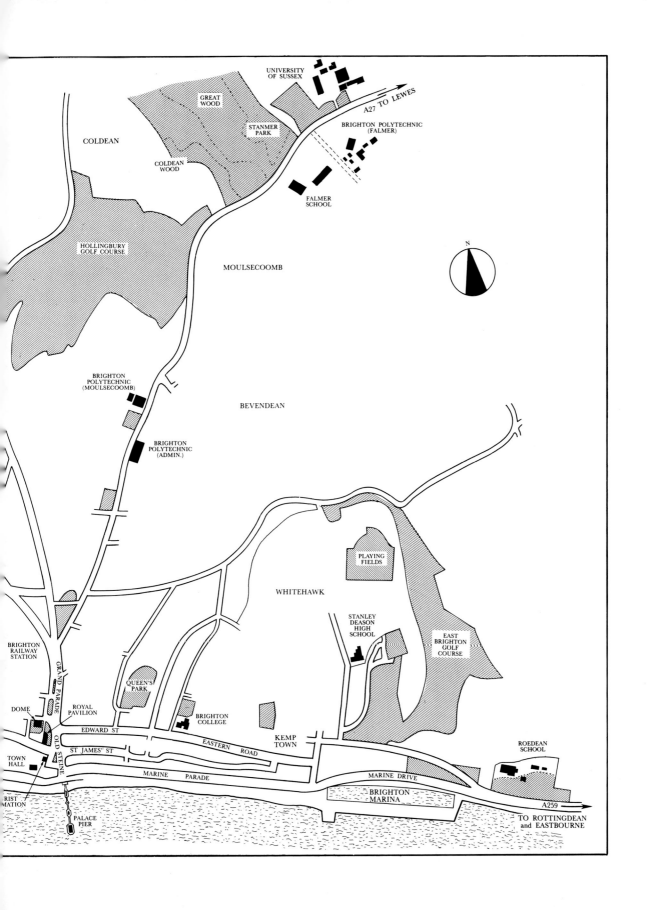